Frederick W.L. Kerr, M.D., is Professor of Neurosurgery and Neuroanatomy, Mayo Foundation and Medical School. In addition, he has written numerous articles on the subject of pain and pain relief.

The Pain Book

FREDERICK W.L. KERR, M.D.
The Mayo Clinic

A SPECTRUM BOOK

Prentice-Hall, Inc.
Englewood Cliffs, New Jersey 07632

Library of Congress Cataloging in Publication Data

KERR, FREDERICK W. L.
The pain book.

(A Spectrum Book)
Includes bibliographies and index.
1. Pain. 2. Pain—Therapy. I. Title.
RB127.K4 616'.0472 81-8653
AACR2

ISBN 0-13-647826-3

ISBN 0-13-647818-2 {PBK.}

10 9 8 7 6 5 4 3 2 1

Editorial/production supervision
and interior design by Eric Newman
Cover design by Honi Werner
Manufacturing buyer: Cathie Lenard

PRENTICE-HALL INTERNATIONAL, INC., *London*
PRENTICE-HALL OF AUSTRALIA PTY. LIMITED, *Sydney*
PRENTICE-HALL OF CANADA, LTD., *Toronto*
PRENTICE-HALL OF INDIA PRIVATE LIMITED, *New Delhi*
PRENTICE-HALL OF JAPAN, INC., *Tokyo*
PRENTICE-HALL OF SOUTHEAST ASIA PTE. LTD., *Singapore*
WHITEHALL BOOKS LIMITED, *Wellington, New Zealand*

Contents

Preface

This book addresses two main aspects of the pain problem. One of these is the general subject of pain as a sensation and as an emotional experience. Some of the issues dealt with in this part of the book are the following: What do we know about the manner in which this unpleasant sensation comes about? Is there a special network of nerve fibers concerned with pain? Are there specific nerve cells and pathways for pain in the brain, and are pain-producing or pain-inhibiting substances released in the body or brain that induce or mitigate pain? Are there great individual differences in tolerance to pain, and if so, why?

The other major issues dealt with are the most pragmatic ones of specific types of pain, such as those of headache, neuralgia, cancer, "slipped disks," and many other common and some less common painful conditions. What causes these pains, and how can we minimize or avoid them? What drugs are really effective for controlling pain and what can be done if they fail? Are there any promising new drugs, and if so, how do they work and are they likely to cause addiction? What can be expected of surgery for pain; should psychosurgery be banned or has it been unjustifiably maligned? Are acupuncture and hypnosis legitimate methods for treating pain, or should they be relegated to the purview of the charlatan or music-hall entertainer?

Because the varieties of pain to which humans are subject is vast, it has been necessary to restrict our discussion to a rather limited number of painful conditions. The selection has been based primarily on two criteria: One of these was the relative frequency of the particular pain problem; in many instances, these painful conditions are introduced with a typical case history. This provides a sense of reality that cannot be achieved by a dry description of symptoms. Sometimes they may help the reader to recognize his own type of pain and to seek appropriate treatment; or they may make it easier to understand the pain of a relative or friend. The other criterion was that the condition, even if rare, illustrated some particular aspect of pain, either because of its intensity or its resistance to treatment and in some instances, because pain cannot be elicited at all!

Two significant areas are not dealt with in any depth, one being that of pains in which psychogenic factors are predominant and the other being the area of malingering or pseudo-pains. Psychogenic factors are of the greatest importance in many pain problems and require the most careful evaluation; however, they have been discussed by many authors in several recent books that have dealt with the subject in considerable detail. I have avoided discussing malingering, or the attempt to derive some pecuniary or psychological advantage from a non-existent, fabricated pain condition; to describe the manner in which the "complaint" is presented or the methods by which the deception can usually be uncovered might provide the malingerer with additional means of evading detection.

Progress in our understanding of pain and the development of improved methods of treatment of painful conditions has depended in good part on advances in knowledge of the neural structures involved. I have addressed this problem in Chapter 2, in which this complex system is described with a minimum of technical terms and with illustrations selected to clarify and emphasize crucial points. An initial version of this section had to be drastically pruned to conform to the publisher's requirements, but I believe that the essential details have been retained.

I have endeavored to correct a number of misconceptions about topics such as psychosurgery, acupuncture, and hypnosis. These areas have been the subject of a great deal of controversy, sometimes entirely justified, but as often based on misinformation. A clear understanding of what is in fact involved and of the shortcomings or benefits that may be expected from these areas of the pain problem may, one hopes, result in more rational dialogues in the future.

ACKNOWLEDGMENTS

I wish to express my indebtedness to a number of people who have contributed by their time, suggestions, and efforts to the outcome of this book.

Dr. Tony L. Yaksh read the chapter on drugs in the treatment of pain, and Dr. Richard W. Marsh read the entire manuscript. To both of them goes my gratitude for their patience and suggestions.

To Sylvia H. Haabala and Patricia J. Erwin (reference) and Ruth J. Mann (history) of the Mayo Clinic Library, for such selfless and very efficient assistance in tracking down references and obtaining copies of reports and portraits of some of the pioneers in the history of research on pain.

To Mary Kennan, editor for Prentice-Hall, Inc., who proposed the project and made many helpful and encouraging suggestions, and to Eric Newman for guiding the book through its vital later stages of production.

Finally, to Ann Rockafellow, my secretary, who uncomplainingly deciphered my manuscript and cheerfully typed and retyped the annotated versions with a minimum of errors and a maximum of efficiency, my lasting appreciation.

1

Dealing with Pain

How we deal with pain is as different as the way we deal with love, play, work, and other challenges of everyday life. True, there are overall similarities in our reactions to each of these situations. It is in the detail, however, where the personal differences are most noticeable, and nowhere is this more apparent than with pain. Take, for example, the experience of having a carious tooth drilled without an anesthetic. As soon as the nerve endings in the tooth are damaged, either mechanically or by the heat generated by the abrasive action of the bit, the most acute pain is felt. The head is jerked away in an involuntary reflex fashion; even with the strongest exercise of willpower, it is difficult for most people to endure this type of pain for more than a few seconds at a time. Associated with the pain, there may be a considerable degree of nervousness and anxiety, sweating and pallor. It is not surprising that visiting the dentist has never been popular, though with the almost universal use of local anesthetics nowadays, the experience has lost most of its old terror.

For a few people, however, the preceding scenario is quite incomprehensible. For them, having a cavity drilled and filled produces little or no discomfort; in fact, they find a local anesthetic more of an inconvenience than an advantage. Yes, they feel pain, and it is apparently quite acute, but it affects them only moderately and is thus quite tolerable. A dentist I knew used to give his services free one afternoon a week to a dental clinic in a port zone. It was not at all uncommon, he informed me, among the many patients he treated for a stevedore to decline any anesthetic, local or otherwise, for an extraction and to tolerate the procedure with little or no signs of pain.

How different was the strapping workman whom I vaccinated against smallpox many years ago. As I approached him with the scarifier, an instrument with a sharp tip used to scrape the skin and allow the vaccine to penetrate, he retreated against the wall and, when he could go no farther, finally submitted. What I was not prepared for was his sudden gasp as the instrument pierced the skin, followed by his precipitate fall to the floor in a dead faint! It was not the pain but the fear of pain that led to his embarrassing collapse. Yet in other circumstances, this man may well have functioned quite admirably.

The rather striking differences in reaction to the pain of childbirth also indicate that pain is not regarded in the same way by all people. For some women, delivery is a frightening, painful, and thoroughly unpleasant experience; for others, profound feelings of emotional fulfillment are so overwhelming that pain and discomfort are relegated to a secondary plane.

Apart from these relatively commonplace types of pain, there are situations in which extremely severe pain is tolerated with a degree of equanimity that is almost unbelievable. Eyewitness accounts of some of these events provide both remarkable testimonials to the fortitude of cer-

Figure 1.1. Surgery before the advent of anesthesia. Baron Dominique Larrey is preparing to amputate the left arm of Captain Rebsomen, who is fully conscious (Battle of Hanau, 1813). Amputation of the arm was followed by amputation of the right leg.
Courtesy of the Musee du Val-de-Grace.

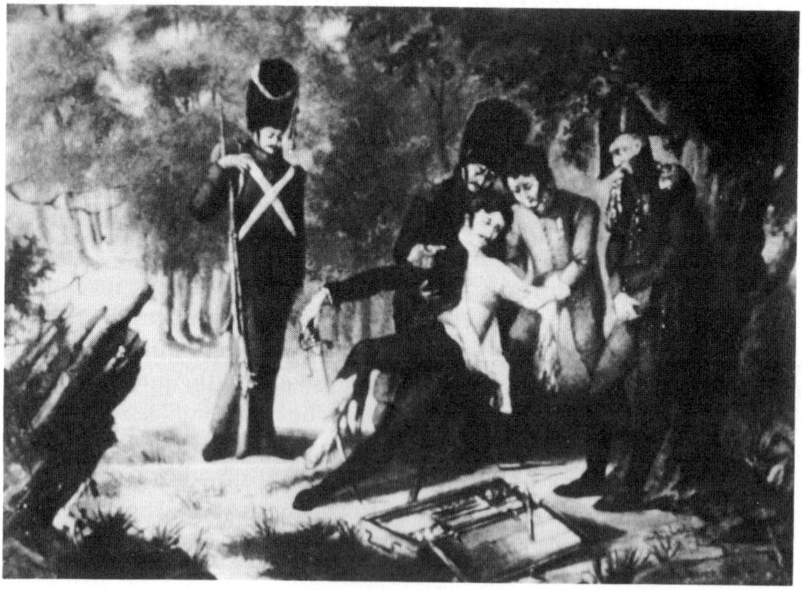

tain individuals and some insight into the complexities of the pain experience. In the reminiscences of some of the great military surgeons of the past, instances of extraordinary fortitude in the face of the most intense pain are frequently recounted. A striking example of this is illustrated in a painting that hangs in the military museum of Val-de-Grace, France, reproduced here by kind permission (Figure 1.1). A young officer, wounded in the battle of Hanau (1813), is about to be operated on by Baron Dominique Larrey, Chief Surgeon of Napoleon's Grande Armée. The officer, Captain Rebsomen, is shown sitting on a drum, his back resting against a comrade. His left arm is shattered from the elbow down and hangs limply in the surgeon's grasp. His right hand rests on the pommel of his sword, while his mangled right leg swings uselessly. Larrey (Figure 1.2) proceeded with deft, swift strokes of his scalpel to sever skin, muscles, arteries, nerves, and, finally, the bone of the arm. The amputation, as was the rule in those days when speed was the only means of reducing the pain of operations, was completed within seconds; it was reported that Larrey could amputate a shoulder in six seconds! The skin was then bound firmly over the stump with bandages fashioned from the patient's own clothes, for Larrey did not use sutures. The surgeon then turned his attention to the officer's right leg, which he amputated just as speedily and skillfully; at the conclusion, the man was evacuated to a nearby village for initial convalescence. What was remarkable about this operation was that not one but two limbs were removed in rapid sequence and that, throughout the entire procedure, the patient remained seated and fully conscious, giving no other evidence of pain than a low groan from time to time. A year later, the officer, with wounds now fully healed, visited Larrey to exhibit the successful result of his treatment.

This is but one recorded example of countless thousands of operations done under the most primitive conditions; certainly, not all of the operations were borne with the same resolution and stoicism, for the records of the period are also full of reports of the cries and groans of the wounded and of patients undergoing surgery; but that many bore it all in silence is well authenticated.

Another celebrated French surgeon, René Leriche (Figure 1.3), whose vast experience and knowledge of pain problems makes him an invaluable and unimpeachable source, recounts some of his experiences as an advisor to the Russian Medical Corps during World War I. He had been demonstrating his techniques for only a few days when, as he describes it:

> At the express request of a group of very aristocratic Russians, who assured me that it was pointless to give certain Cossacks an anesthetic, since they felt nothing, I proceeded, with no little repugnance, to amputate three fingers and their corresponding metacarpals in one Cossack, and the entire foot of

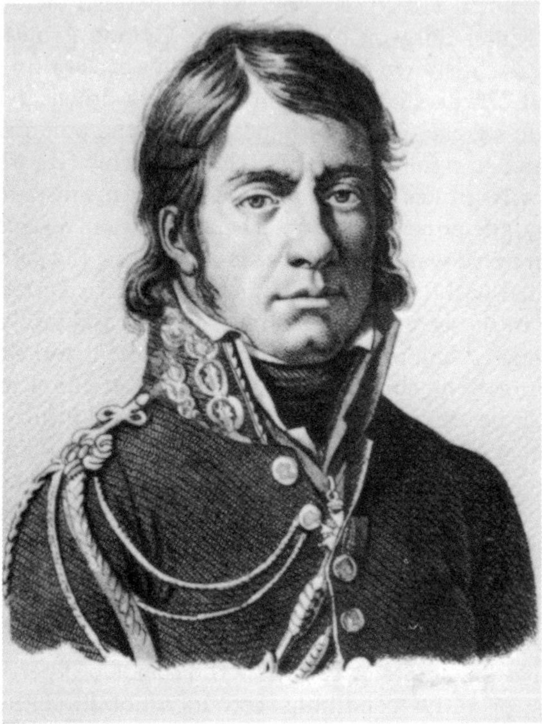

Figure 1.2. Dominique Jean, First Baron Larrey (1766–1842).
Born of sturdy peasant stock at Beaudeau in the French Pyrenees, Larrey attended the Toulouse School of Medicine and Surgery. At fifteen he was already a surgical "dresser," advancing to house surgeon before graduating in 1786. While in Paris in 1789, he took care of some of the injured in the assault on the Bastille. He became a military surgeon in Napoleon's army and rapidly rose to the rank of professor of surgery at the military hospital of Val-de-Grace.

A man of immense energy and great strength—he claimed to be the strongest man in Napoleon's army—he participated in nearly all the major battles, including the Russian campaign. Operating under appalling conditions with the temperature often at or below freezing, he was still able to save the lives of 75 percent of the patients who underwent amputations, whereas other surgeons of the period saved only 10 percent.

Larrey can probably be regarded as the greatest military surgeon of all time. Not only was he a technical virtuoso who could amputate a hip in thirteen seconds (at Borodino he performed 200 amputations in twenty-four hours), but he so improved the field ambulance service that at Aboukir, none of the French wounded waited more than forty-five minutes for treatment. And his methods of treatment anticipated developments by a century and more.

Portrait courtesy of the National Library of Medicine.

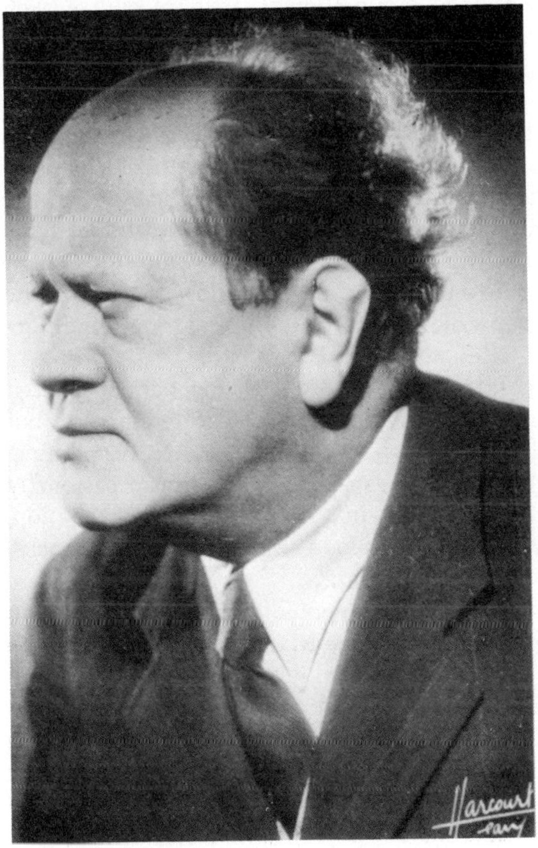

Figure 1.3. René Leriche (1879–1955).
The son of a lawyer, Leriche was born at Roanne in central France. He was graduated from the medical school at Lyons in 1906, and in 1920 he was appointed to the school's chair of experimental surgery. In 1924, he became Professor of Clinical Surgery at Strasbourg, and in 1937 he won the coveted chair of medicine at the College de France, Paris. For a quarter of a century he was the leading surgical figure in Europe and received virtually every honor of significance in his field. He was described by his colleagues as modest and unassuming and was esteemed as much for his originality of thought as for his surgical judgment and skill. His numerous contributions to the literature were distinguished by their solid basis in physiology and their correlation with clinical-surgical problems. In addition to his major treatise on pain (*La Chirurgie de la Douleur,* 1937), he wrote books on subjects as diverse as the physiology and pathology of bone and the disorders of blood vessels.

Illustration reprinted by permission from *Journal of Cardiovascular Surgery* 1: 233, 1960.

> another. Neither man so much as quivered, turning the hand or raising the leg at my request without faltering for an instant, as if they had been under the most perfect of local anesthetics. [Author's translation]

In this episode, it is important to note that Leriche makes the point that only *certain* Cossacks appeared to feel no pain; thus, this behavioral characteristic was not common to the Russian troops as a whole but only to a very limited and racially defined group thereof. It is, of course, well known that certain races, from antiquity to the present, have exhibited, either collectively or in a significant proportion of their number, a most surprising ability to endure pain without manifesting any signs of discomfort. Among the ancients, the Spartans were renowned for their hardiness and contempt for comfort. Of the many stories told of their legendary stoicism, perhaps none illustrates this quality more graphically than the possibly apocryphal account of a youth who had hidden a fox beneath his gown in defiance of his elders. Rather than be discovered, he stood silent and unflinching as it ripped his belly open. Little wonder that the name *Spartan* to this day conjures up visions of fortitude, courage, and indifference to pain.

During the Middle Ages, the religious order of flagellants chastised themselves unmercifully with knouts (whips made of knotted thongs), but no complaint passed their lips as they silently threaded their way among awe-stricken spectators; even today, newspaper photographs occasionally appear of individuals in Eastern countries in a state of religious exaltation, flogging themselves with chains until the blood streams down their backs, yet they show no outward signs of suffering!

A particularly striking and well-documented example of stoicism in this continent concerns the young men of the Mandan Indian tribe in the Dakota territories who had to prove their manliness by bearing mutilation and torture without complaint, during the celebration of the summer festival of O-kee-pa. George Catlin (1796–1872), artist and chronicler of the Old West, was permitted to witness this gruesome ceremony during a tour of the Dakotas in 1833. His vivid portrayal of the scene (Figure 1.4) is an authentic record not only of tribal customs but of human endurance under extreme conditions of pain and suffering.

Catlin described the ceremony as follows:

> . . . two men, having taken their positions near the middle of the lodge, for the purpose of inflicting the tortures—the one with the scalping-knife, and the other with the bunch of splints (which I have before mentioned) in his hand; one at a time [one] of the young fellows, already emaciated with fasting, and thirsting, and waking, for nearly four days and nights, advanced from the side of the lodge, and placed himself on his hands and feet, or otherwise, as best suited for the performance of the operation, where he

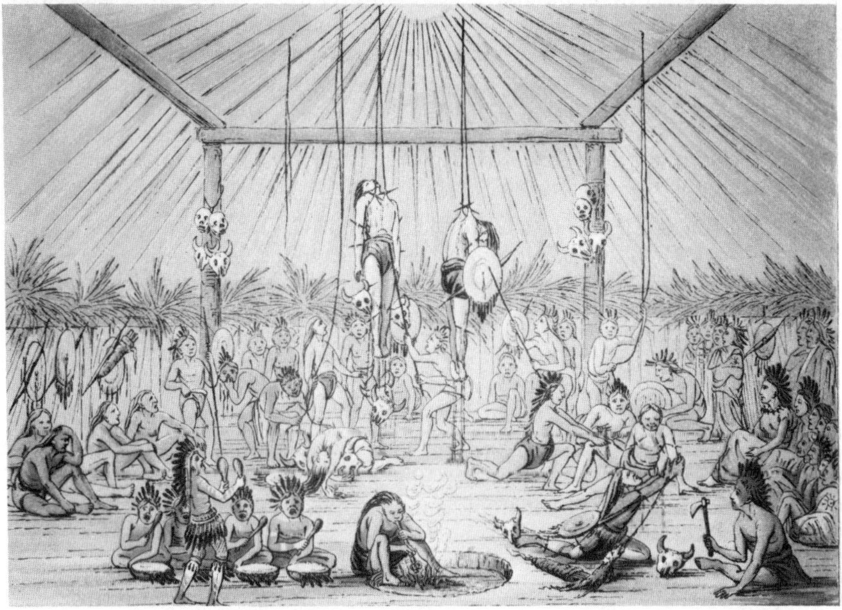

Figure 1.4. O-kee-pa ceremony of the Mandan tribe. The candidate braves are shown at several stages in the initiation rites; note the heavy buffalo skulls and other weights attached to the hanging men, a brave rotating one of the candidates with a spear (center left), and the candidate preparing to offer his finger to be chopped by the elder (lower right).
From George Catlin, *Illustrations of the Manners, Customs and Conditions of the North American Indians* (Vol. I). Piccadilly, London: Chatto and Windus, pp. 170–172.

submitted to the cruelties in the following manner: An inch or more of the flesh on each shoulder, or each breast, was taken up between the thumb and finger by the man who held the knife in his right hand; and the knife, which had been ground sharp on both edges, and then hacked and notched with the blade of another, to make it produce as much pain as possible, was forced through the flesh below the fingers, and, being withdrawn, was followed with a splint or skewer, from the other, who held a bunch of such in his left hand, and was ready to force them through the wound. There were then two cords lowered down from the top of the lodge (by men who were placed on the lodge outside, for the purpose), which were fastened to these splints or skewers, and they instantly began to haul him up; he was thus raised until his body was suspended from the ground where he rested, until the knife and a splint were passed through the flesh or integuments in a similar manner on each arm below the shoulder (over the brachialis externus), below the elbow (over the extensor carpi radialis), on the thighs (over the vastus externus), and below the knees (over the peroneus).

In some instances they remained in a reclining position on the ground until this painful operation was finished, which was performed, in all instances, exactly on the same parts of the body and limbs; and which, in its progress, occupied some five or six minutes.

Each one was then instantly raised with the cords, until the weight of his body was suspended by them, and then, while the blood was streaming down their limbs, the bystanders hung upon the splints each man's appropriate shield, bow and quiver, &c.; and in many instances, the skull of a buffalo with the horns on it, was attached to each lower arm and each lower leg, for the purpose, probably, of preventing by their great weight, the struggling, which might otherwise have taken place to their disadvantage whilst they were hung up.

When these things were all adjusted, each one was raised higher by the cords, until these weights all swung clear from the ground, leaving his feet, in most cases, some six or eight feet above the ground. In this plight they at once became appalling and frightful to look at—the flesh, to support the weight of their bodies, with the additional weights which were attached to them, was raised six or eight inches by the skewers; and their heads sunk forward on the breasts, or thrown backwards, in a much more frightful condition, according to the way in which they were hung up.

The unflinching fortitude with which every one of them bore this part of the torture surpassed credulity; each one as the knife was passed through his flesh sustained an unchangeable countenance; and several of them, seeing me making sketches, beckoned me to look at their faces, which I watched through all this horrid operation, without being able to detect anything but the pleasantest smiles as they looked me in the eye, while I could hear the knife rip through the flesh, and feel enough of it myself, to start involuntary and uncontroullable [*sic*] tears over my cheeks.

When [they were] raised to the condition above described, and completely suspended by the cords, the sanguinary hands, through which he had just passed, turned back to perform a similar operation on another who was ready, and each one in his turn passed into the charge of others, who instantly introduced him to a new and improved state of their refinements in cruelty.

Surrounded by imps and demons as they appear, a dozen or more, who seem to be concerting and devising means for his exquisite agony, gather around him, when one of the number advances towards him in a sneering manner, and commences turning him around with a pole which he brings in his hand for the purpose. This is done in a gentle manner at first; but gradually increased, when the brave fellow, whose proud spirit can control its agony no longer, burst out in the most lamentable and heart-rending cries that the human voice is capable of producing, crying forth a prayer to the Great Spirit to support and protect him in this dreadful trial; and continually repeating his confidence in his protection. In this condition he is continued to be turned, faster and faster—and there is no hope of escape from it, nor chance for the slightest relief, until by fainting, his voice falters, and his struggling ceases, and he hangs, apparently, a still and lifeless corpse! When he is, by turning, gradually brought to this condition, which is generally done within ten or fifteen minutes, there is a close scrutiny passed upon him among his tormentors, who are checking and holding each other back as long as the least struggling or tremour [*sic*] can be discovered, lest he should be removed before he is (as they term it) "entirely dead."

> When brought to this alarming and most frightful condition, and the turning has gradually ceased, as his voice and his strength have given out, leaving him to hang entirely still, and apparently lifeless; when his tongue is distended from his mouth, and his *medicine-bag*, which he has affectionately and superstitiously clung to with his left hand, has dropped to the ground; the signal is given to the men on top of the lodge, by gently striking the cord with the pole below, when they very gradually and carefully lower him to the ground.
>
> In this helpless condition he lies, like a loathsome corpse to look at, though in the keeping (as they call it) of the Great Spirit, who he trusts will protect him, and enable him to get up and walk away. As soon as he is lowered to the ground thus, one of the bystanders advances, and pulls out the two splints or pins from the breasts and shoulders, thereby disengaging him from the cords by which he has been hung up; but leaving all the others with their weights, &c. hanging to his flesh.
>
> In this condition he lies for six or eight minutes, until he gets strength to rise and move himself, for no one is allowed to assist or offer him aid, as he is here enjoying the most valued privilege which a Mandan can boast of, that of "trusting his life to the keeping of the Great Spirit," in this time of extreme peril.
>
> As soon as he is seen to get strength enough to rise on his hands and feet, and drag his body around the lodge, he crawls with the weithts still hanging to his body, to another part of the lodge, where there is another Indian sitting with a hatchet in his hand, and a dried buffalo skull before him; and here, in the most earnest and humble manner, by holding up the little finger of his left hand to the Great Spirit, he expresses to Him, in a speech of a few words, his willingness to give it as a sacrifice; when he lays it on the dried buffalo skull, where the other chops it off near the hand, with a blow of the hatchet!
>
> Nearly all of the young men whom I saw passing this horrid ordeal gave, in the above manner, the little finger of the left hand; and I saw also several, who immediately afterwards (and apparently with very little concern or emotion), with a similar speech, extended in the same way, the forefinger of the same hand, and that too was struck off; leaving on the left hand only the two middle fingers and the thumb; all which they deem absolutely essential for holding the bow, the only weapon for the left hand.

Once six or eight candidates had completed this ordeal, they were taken outside, still loaded down with the weights hanging from the skewers in their flesh and dragging on the ground. Two powerful braves then secured their wrists with broad leather straps and, grasping them by these, rushed around an altar in the center of the encampment, dragging the tortured, stumbling candidate behind them. Finally, he would again faint and fall to the ground as if dead; and then, semiconscious, with his face in the dirt, he was dragged around furiously until the weights tore the skewers out of his flesh. This final part of the ceremony was aptly known as the "Last

Race"; he then had to drag himself unassisted back to his own lodge. The ordeal was over; he was now a Mandan brave!

The foregoing is but a short summary of some of the better authenticated instances of unusual tolerance to pain. I have not discussed the spectacular feats of Indian fakirs who transfix their cheeks and other parts of their anatomy with needles, nor the fire walkers and other sensational performers. In some instances it is probable that the individual is suffering from disorders such as neural leprosy or syringomyelia, in which case he would feel no pain, as described in Chapter 8. Others may be in a state of religious exaltation, akin perhaps to self-hypnosis. Of course, the ever-present possibility of deception must be kept in mind.

WHY SUCH STRIKING DIFFERENCES?

The gap that separates the response of a Cossack who allows his foot to be amputated with apparent complete indifference to pain from that of the person who cries out in anguish when pricked with a sharp hypodermic needle is evidently enormous. How can we account for a spectrum so broad, ranging from the stoic at one end to the pusillanimous at the other?

The first and simplest answer is that individual sensitivity to pain must vary strikingly. But what precisely do we mean by sensitivity? We could be thinking about the ability to perceive pain as sensation. To give a comparison, the ability to hear very high frequency tones varies considerably and decreases with the passage of years. In the case of pain, the actual point at which one perceives that a stimulus has passed from being comfortable to being painful, or what is termed the *pain threshold*, is very similar from person to person.

Numerous methods of determining pain thresholds have been devised beginning with von Frey in Germany at the end of the last century. In the 1940s, H. Wolff and associates introduced the radiant heat method, in which a beam of hot light was focused on a patch of skin that had been blackened for maximal absorption. A scale of pain intensities extending from threshold to maximum tolerated and divided into twenty successive increments in intensity, designated as dols (from the Latin *dolor,* or pain), was established. Test subjects were able to discriminate the twenty stepwise increases with considerable accuracy. When the skin is heated to temperatures of up to 44° centigrade, subjects report heat but not pain. At or around 45° C, the sensation changes more or less rapidly to frank pain; and as the temperature is increased a degree at a time, the degree of discomfort soom becomes intolerable, and the stimulated area is withdrawn sharply. What is especially significant is that the great majority of persons tested for response to heat perceive the transition to pain (the threshold for pain) at or very close to the same temperature. It is, of course, important to take into account skin thickness, as on the soles of the feet, and adaptation to handling hot tools (cooks, welders, and so on).

The pain threshold is very similar not only among people of the same race but from one race to another, and even from humans to other mammals such as the dog, cat, and rat, provided, of course, that skin areas of comparable thickness are tested. However, the response to pain at higher intensities varies to a very significant degree among individuals and groups.

In a recent study in which electrical stimulation of the skin was used, Clark and associates (1980) compared pain responses in Nepalese porters with those of Westerners in a field study, in view of criticisms that have been leveled at results obtained in a laboratory environment. They found that both groups identified the sensory phenomenon of pain at the same level—that is, perception of threshold was identical—but the reporting of pain, especially of higher intensities, was very much lower in the Nepalese than in the Westerners. They attributed this difference, as had others in comparable circumstances previously, to the greater stoicism of a hardier group of people.

From this and from what I have said about pain perception, it is obvious that all people who exhibit extraordinary stoicism feel pain and that much if not all of that pain must have fallen in the category that most people would regard as intolerable—that is, in the mid to upper range of the dol scale. Yet they showed little or no evidence that they were suffering. This being the case, the only reasonable conclusion would seem to be that the emotional response or expression of pain is radically different in certain people. If this is the explanation, why should emotional factors be so remarkably different?

Experience and Training

That experiences during early development may have a profound influence on subsequent behavior patterns cannot be questioned. In the case of pain, there is both factual and anecdotal evidence to support this assertion. A most striking experimental demonstration of the influence of experience on pain behavior was devised by Ronald Melzack and T. H. Scott of the Department of Psychology at McGill University, Montreal, Canada. The objective of the experiment was to raise dogs from birth in a protected and isolated environment, so that their behavior patterns would not be influenced in any way by observation of older animals who had already acquired "experience." When these "restricted" animals were confronted as adults with the usual or "normal" environment, their behavior was remarkably inappropriate, especially where responses to pain-producing stimuli were concerned.

When they were shown a lighted match, they approached it without fear, nuzzled it, and sometimes snuffed it out by sniffing at it. Not only did they give no signs of having felt pain, but they returned and repeated the process. At the time, it was midwinter in Montreal, and, incredibly, these dogs would repeatedly lick extremely hot central-heating pipes without evincing any signs of pain. In striking contrast to normal control dogs, the "restricted" dogs not only showed highly inappropriate responses to noxious stimuli, but they rarely if ever yelped when injured and, futhermore, showed little or no tendency to learn to avoid damaging situations; even after two years of unrestricted existence, some dogs continued to exhibit almost identically defective behavior. The role of learning in the expression of emotional responses is singularly well brought out by this simple yet elegant experiment.

The influence of learning on the interpretation of events is profoundly and irreversibly affected in other sensory systems. I refer in particular to vision in children who are born with a congenital cataract. When this is removed at a later date, though light perception is retained in the affected eye, ability to recognize objects is never regained. From this, it appears reasonably clear that there is a "training period" when the brain is young and its connections are still very malleable. If training does not take place during this critical period, the right connections fail to occur, and no amount of subsequent exercise or practice can make up for the lost opportunity.

Although these fundamental processes of maturation of brain circuitry leading to recognition occur during infancy, additional and important learning processes occur throughout childhood and, with diminishing effectiveness, in adult life. What better evidence of this do we need than the commonplace observation that languages are learned with greater facility by the young and that excellence in most sports requiring skill, such as figure skating, tennis, and other ball games, demands intensive early training. Certainly, an adult can learn to perform in any of these spheres with an acceptable degree of expertise, but it is rare indeed that such late starters achieve championship form. It is not farfetched, therefore, to suggest by analogy that patterns of behavioral response to pain learned in childhood will determine, to a significant or major degree, the adult's emotional reactions to pain. The child who observes parents and other adults behaving in a highly emotional way in response to minor injuries can be expected to behave in a like manner when he or she is similarly injured. Conversely, in a social environment in which injuries are borne with relative indifference, and especially, when any display of emotion is strongly discouraged and disapproved, the responses are much more likely to be stoical in the face of pain. Thus, the pain may be felt with similar intensity by the great majority, but whereas the emotional expression of suffering is florid in one group, it is negligible or absent in another. Some of the examples of exceptional fortitude toward pain referred to earlier can be considered again in the light of these observations.

How can we account for the striking disparities in the respective attitudes and responses of Spartans and Athenians to discomfort, pain, and suffering? Clearly, the major and possibly the only factor that we can pinpoint is the profound difference in upbringing. The Spartan child was trained from the age of five or six to endure physical hardship without complaint; it was a matter of honor and pride to bear pain and discomfort unflinchingly. The Athenians, on the other hand, put much less stock in such stoical virtues; it is not surprising that their descendants were not renowned for any particular qualities of hardiness. Similarly, the Cossacks have a long tradition of showing indifference to physical suffering, their children being raised in accord with strict precepts of endurance and stoicism. To this point, the discussion of human response to pain and suffering supports the thesis that experience and training are the determining factors in the differences observed. At least, no better explanation appears available.

However, can we go any further and at least try to suggest additional bases for these marked divergences in behavioral response? In what way can training so alter an important and highly structured neural apparatus? In addition to the anatomical deficits that appear to occur, are there also physiological or biochemical changes of sufficient magnitude that enable an appropriately trained individual to allow his unanesthetized foot to be amputated without a murmur of complaint?

We do not as yet have any factual answers to this question, but recent advances in our knowledge of the structure and function of the central nervous system and of pain mechanisms permit some speculative suggestions. There is both structural and physiological evidence now that the connections established by certain circuits in the brain are considerably less immutable than had previously been supposed. This is true not only for the immature brain (i.e., of the newborn) but also for some adult systems and especially for some species such as the rat. It is probable that training and practice may subtly modify central networks to some extent; this line of investigation is still at an early stage, and much will be learned in the coming decade.

What is the likelihood that biochemical changes may be produced by the learning process? Here the probabilities are even higher, but it must always be remembered that we are still dealing with probability and not established fact. This caveat having been made, we can now permit ourselves the luxury of speculating.

Enkephalin and endorphins, naturally occurring and potent painkillers (Chapter 10), are manufactured and released in many areas of the brain. Why the brain produces these substances is not known, nor do we know under what circumstances they are released. However, the very fact that they are present, and that their analgesic potency is similar to that of morphine, can lead us to ask whether their levels may vary considerably from one person to another and within a given person at various times.

If this hypothesis were to be proven, then many of our questions about the vagaries of pain might be explained. Thus, it is conceivable that an individual who begins at an early age to suppress his or her emotional reactions to pain may, in fact, be learning to activate nerve networks in the brain that either produce or release stored enkephalin. As a result, such people who have temporarily "flooded" their pain circuits with enkephalin might be far better able to tolerate severe pain. Conversely, some people may have relatively scanty stores of enkephalin or may be less able to release it on demand; the consequence of such a defect would presumably be a greater sensitivity to pain and, attached thereto, the stigma of being pusillanimous.

It is also quite conceivable that long-continued or chronic pain may lead either to the depletion of normal reserves of enkephalin or, more likely, to the development of a tolerance to it; in either case, the behavioral result would be more pain, more suffering, and more complaints. However, when this interesting hypothesis was tested by Lindblom and Tegner (1979), no evidence could be found to support it.

Are some of the pale, anguished, chronically complaining patients seen in the outpatient departments of all hospitals actually people who have a deficit of endorphins? Some evidence for this has been provided by von Knorring et al. (1978), who found significant differences in the levels of endorphin in the spinal fluid of patients with chronic pain; higher levels of endorphins correlated with increased threshold and greater tolerance to electrically evoked pain. It is just possible that we have done some chronic complainers an injustice by too lightly dismissing their complaints as imaginary. Did some of them actually have a deficit of endorphins?

We might, futhermore, remember that the very existence of endorphins and enkephalins was not even suspected a decade ago, yet they are now central to any discussion of pain mechanisms. Are there other naturally occurring modulating substances, with perhaps equal or greater actions on pain, that are yet to be discovered? If so, perhaps many of the problems alluded to in this chapter might be clarified and speculation laid to rest.

REFERENCES

CATLIN, GEORGE. *Illustrations of the Manners, Customs and Condition of the North American Indians* (Vol. I). Piccadilly, London: Chatto and Windus, pp. 170–172.

CLARK, W.C., and CLARK, S.B. Pain response in Nepalese porters. *Science* 209: 410–412, 1980.

KNORRING, L. VON; ALMAY, B.G.L.; JOHANSSON, F.; and TERENIUS, L. Pain perception and endorphin levels in spinal fluid. *Pain* 5: 359–365, 1978.

LERICHE, RENÉ. *La chirurgie de la douleur.* Paris: Masson et Cie., 1937, 428 pp.

LINDBLOM, U., and TEGNER, R. Are the endorphins active in clinical pain states? Narcotic antagonism in chronic-pain patients. *Pain* 7: 65–68, 1979.

MELZACK, R., and SCOTT, T.H. The effects of early experience on the response to pain. *Journal of Comparative Psychology* 50: 155–161, 1957.

Structural and functional evidence of plasticity in the central nervous system. *Experimental Neurology* 48: 16–31, 1975 (Ed. by F.W.L. Kerr).

WOLFF, B.B. Measurement of human pain. In Pain, *Assn. R.N.M.D.* Vol. 58: 173–184 (Ed. by J.J. Bonica). New York: Raven Press, 1980.

WOLFF, H.G.; HARDY, J.D.; and GOODELL, H. Studies in pain: discrimination of differences in intensity of painful stimuli. Transactions of the American Neurological Association 71: 163–164, 1946.

2

Nerves, the Brain, and Pain

Someone has said that the brain is the most complex system in the universe. Hyperbole—or possibly just another of those all-too-common overstatements designed to catch the eye? In this instance, the comparison may not be so farfetched; consider the following facts uncovered by past and contemporary neuroscientists, keeping in mind that they are cautious and relatively conservative conclusions.

The nervous system is composed of myriad nerve cells, technically referred to as *neurons*. Although neurons come in an almost infinite variety of shapes, in general they can be regarded as having a body, or *soma* (spherical, elongated, pyramid-shaped, or other), from which arise a number of fine filaments. One of these, known as the *axon*, plays a major role in communication in that it serves to conduct impulses from one cell body to another. The other processes, or *dendrites*, are usually shorter and can be regarded as collecting elements that receive messages from other neurons and conduct them toward their parent cell body.

Until approximately 1970, it was commonly stated that there were some 10 billion of these neurons in the human cerebral cortex alone, but more recent research has shown quite conclusively that this number is closer to 50 billion and that another 40 billion neurons are to be found in the cortex of the cerebellum. It is probable, therefore, that there are more than 100 billion neurons in the entire human nervous system, a prodigious and totally incomprehensible figure.

Impressive as these numbers are, they are but a surface indicator of an even greater complexity. As noted earlier, neurons communicate with each other by means of an axon. This extremely slender filament, on reaching its target, usually breaks up into a number of fine terminal branches, each of which ends with a tiny bulbous swelling known as the *bouton*, or end bulb. The number of end bulbs stemming from a given axon ranges from some half dozen to as many as 100 thousand or more. The point of contact between these terminals and their target cell is called a *synapse*.

To sum up, there are some 100 billion neurons capable of making synaptic contacts between one another by means of tens or even hundreds of thousands of terminals. Next to this, the most complex computer yet developed appears to be but a child's toy. Need one be reminded that the computer was conceived by the human brain?

Another remarkable feature of the brain is that this infinitely complex system is not, as one might imagine upon looking at specially prepared sections under a microscope, an inextricable or haphazard tangle of cells, fibers, and endings. To the contrary, it is organized in the most exquisitely perfect manner; each ending, or set of endings, terminates on a specified target cell. Even this termination is in no way haphazard, for during brain development, in some inexplicable manner, the endings found their way to specific sites on the target cells, where they established their definitive contacts.

We should remember, too, that this complex organ is turned out daily by the hundreds of thousands, each an almost perfect replica of every other one and thus indistinguishable even under the microscope or the electron microscope. Yet any one of them may carry within it the potential for that vast range of human activities that extends from athletic prowess to artistic and intellectual accomplishments of the highest order; and each brain will express itself with a different personality and a different set of emotional responses. Somehow, 100 billion neurons "know" how to get together and organize themselves into that most perfect of organs, the human brain; unlike machines, most of them function perfectly for decades and occasionally for as long as a century!

THE BRAIN AND PAIN

Of all the innumerable functions carried out by the brain, the one that is the subject of this book occupies a most important place. As we shall see, our very survival depends on the warnings that the defense systems in the brain provide when our bodily integrity is threatened. How this part of the brain is structured and how it functions is still imperfectly understood. In the following paragraphs, a very condensed version of this basic aspect of p ain is given; for the reader seeking more information, references at the end of the chapter provide leads to the scientific literature.

Before dealing with these issues, it is necessary to comment, albeit briefly, on some concepts of pain and on the semantic and scientific difficulties that confront those who attempt to deal with the subject.

Pain as a Sensation

Because it is difficult to define *pain,* the usual response to this issue has been to use a more or less synonymous term, such as *hurt* or *unpleasant sensation*.

Sir Charles S. Sherrington (1857–1952), the English physiologist, emphasized the cardinal fact that pain develops when tissue integrity is threatened. Although exceptions to this rule exist, it is a basic factor in all pain-related situations.

Whether pain should be considered a separate sensation or simply an exaggeration of other basic sensory modalities, such as pressure or heat, for example, is an issue that was debated for many years. With the introduction of more sophisticated techniques for recording from nerve fibers and cells, the predominantly theoretical and philosophical discussions of the past began to lose ground and were progressively replaced by scientific observations and hypotheses. A careful evaluation of the situation was made in 1971 by E. R. Perl, the neurophysiologist, in an article entitled "Is Pain a Separate Sensation?" His conclusion, based on electrophysiological and other data, was that the time had come to give tentative recognition to pain as a separate sensation. This view has gained ground steadily during the ensuing decade, and it is probably safe to state that the majority of investigators and physicians concerned with pain so regard it at this time.

THE CONCEPT OF NOCICEPTION

The experience that we call *pain* involves a number of aspects, from the sensory message in the periphery until it reaches a conscious level, together with the variable emotional response it evokes.

One of the issues raised about pain concerns the moment at which a message that is signaling damage ceases to be just a signal and should be regarded as the sensation (pain). To circumvent this difficulty, the neutral term *nociceptive* was introduced to designate activity that was related to, or produced by, a damaging stimulus. Thus, after an injury to a limb, for example, more or less intense neural activity is engendered in the nerve fibers in the skin, but no one would claim that pain was being felt in the skin. The impulses are then transmitted along the nerves; once again, pain is not felt *in* the nerves. The term *nociceptive* was devised to describe such signals; it means simply that noxious stimuli are being received or transmitted. The exact level such messages must reach in the brain before pain is perceived is still uncertain. Some believe that it occurs only when the *thalamus* is reached; others, that it may first appear somewhat lower in the brain, in the area known as the *midbrain*. (See the Glossary for explanations of these terms.)

Reception and the Conduction of Nociceptive Signals

Specialized receptor cells have been developed by the various sensory systems to transform physical events from the environment into electrical signals that can then be relayed by the nerves. The retinal rods and cones and the hair cells of the inner ear are examples; these are transducers of physical stimuli into electrical signals, and the information they collect from the outside world is relayed to consciousness by nerve cells.

Pain, on the other hand, differs from the other sensations in that there are no specialized transducer cells in sites from which pain can be elicited—only free nerve endings. How noxious stimuli activate the free nerve endings is still unknown. The most common proposals entail the release by the damaging agent of a substance such as histamine, bradykinin, potassium, serotonin, prostaglandins, or substance P. All of these can be extracted from damaged tissues, and except for substance P, they produce pain when injected into normal skin. However, it has been difficult to demonstrate in a convincing manner a direct cause-and-effect relationship between any of them and pain.

In recent years, the introduction of extremely sensitive techniques for demonstrating the presence of peptides in tissues has enabled Thomas Hökfelt and his colleagues of the Karolinska Institute in Stockholm to show that substance P is precisely where it would be expected in skin and in certain centers in the brain, if indeed it is responsible for the activation of pain endings. Although it is not yet possible to claim that substance P is the elusive "pain transmitter substance," at this time it appears to be the most likely candidate. It is good to remember, also, that more than one pain transmitter may be required for different types of pain. As noted later, prostaglandins probably play a very important role in certain painful states; the relief of pain by drugs such as aspirin and zomepirac (Zomax) which inhibit the synthesis of prostaglandins, is persuasive evidence in this respect (see Chapter 10).

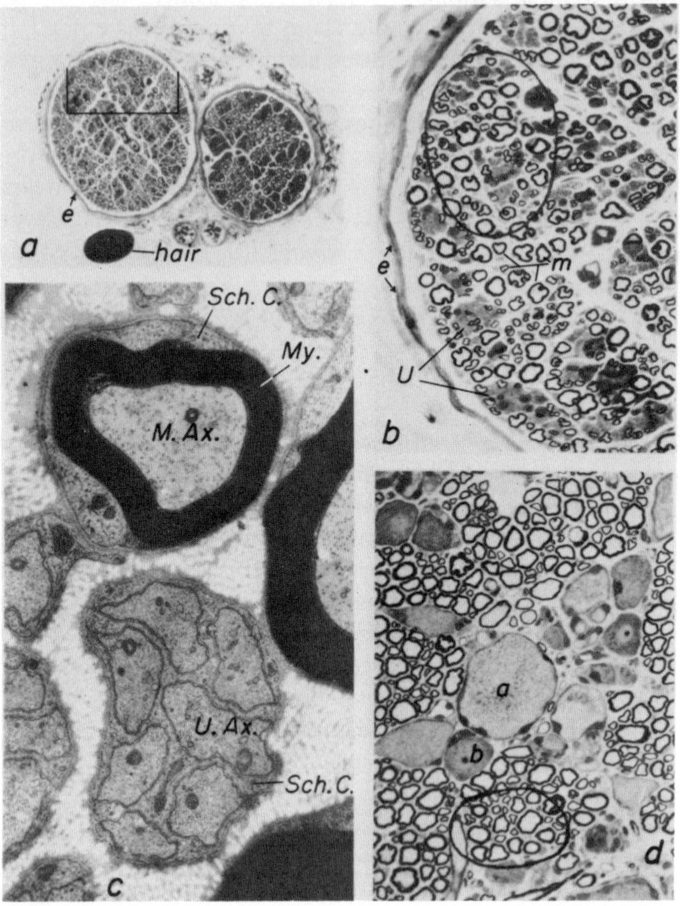

Figure 2.1. *(a)* Two fine branches to the skin from a sensory nerve (saphenous) in the leg (Mag. 135X). The larger branch measured 0.3 mm in diameter and contained close to 1000 myelinated fibers. The dark oval profile beside it and the oval outlines in *(b)* and *(d)* represent an identically cut and processed human hair (diameter 60 μm), providing a more objective idea of the magnifications used.

(b) At higher magnification (540X), the myelinated fibers are seen to range from 9 μm down to 1μm; 70 myelinated fibers are encompassed within the oval profile. However, much smaller fibers are to be found in the apparently structureless gray islets scattered throughout; these are the unmyelinated axons, which are seen well only with the electron microscope, as in *(c)*.

(c) At this magnification (24,000X), the diameter of a hair would be just under 1.5 meters (5 ft.). The diameter of the small myelinated fiber (M.Ax.) is 2 μm; beneath it is a cluster of seven unmyelinated fibers whose transverse diameters range from 0.5 *(b)* to 0.3 *(c)*.

(d) Section through a dorsal root ganglion showing large *(a)* and small *(b)* nerve cells from which the sensory nerve fibers stem (330X).

PERIPHERAL NERVES AND PAIN

The fine free nerve endings in skin and other tissues that are activated by pain-producing injuries are terminals of fibers in the peripheral nerves. Figure 2.1 illustrates what a peripheral nerve looks like at various magnifications when cut across and appropriately stained for observation with the light or electron microscope. Because the conventional calibration mark—a bar indicating a certain number of microns (thousandths of a millimeter)—may convey little to those who are unaccustomed to microscopy, I have substituted a cross section of a human hair, photographed at the same magnification, in each instance. Hairs measure 60 microns in their greater diameter and, interestingly, are oval in cross section.

Photomicrograph 2.1(*a*) shows cross sections of two fine cutaneous nerves; a tough fibrous capsule, the *epineurium*, surrounds large numbers of fine tubules, the *nerve fibers*, some of which can just be made out at this magnification. The succeeding photomicrographs are taken at progressively greater magnification; some idea of the miniaturization involved may be gained from the fact that 100 or more nerve fibers can fit comfortably within the cross-sectional area of a single hair. Perhaps even more remarkable is the fact that these vanishingly fine threads, far thinner than the strands of a spider's web, function perfectly for decades despite the fact that during normal activity, they are subjected to mechanical stresses—such as pressure, stretch, and contusion—that might be expected to damage them beyond repair. When such injury occurs and the nerve is severely contused or transected, the distal part of the axon dies off and degenerates, but this eventuality can also be remedied. From the surviving central stump of the nerve fiber, a sprout appears that grows peripherally along the remains of the degenerated nerve until it reaches the skin, muscle, or other target, where it proceeds to reinnervate it! Admittedly, the restoration of function is rarely perfect, but the fact that regeneration occurs at all is surprising enough. It should be noted that regenerative phenomena also occur in the central nervous system but are much less pronounced and probably never reestablish normal function.

Myelinated and Unmyelinated Axons

Specialized elements called *Schwann cells* wrap themselves around axons from a few times for those of smaller diameter to twenty or thirty times in those of large caliber. This creates a sheath, which is of multilayered appearance when seen at high magnification, that is termed *myelin.* This myelin sheath is not continuous, however, but forms a series of cylindrical cuffs; think of an electric wire in which the insulation is interrupted by a

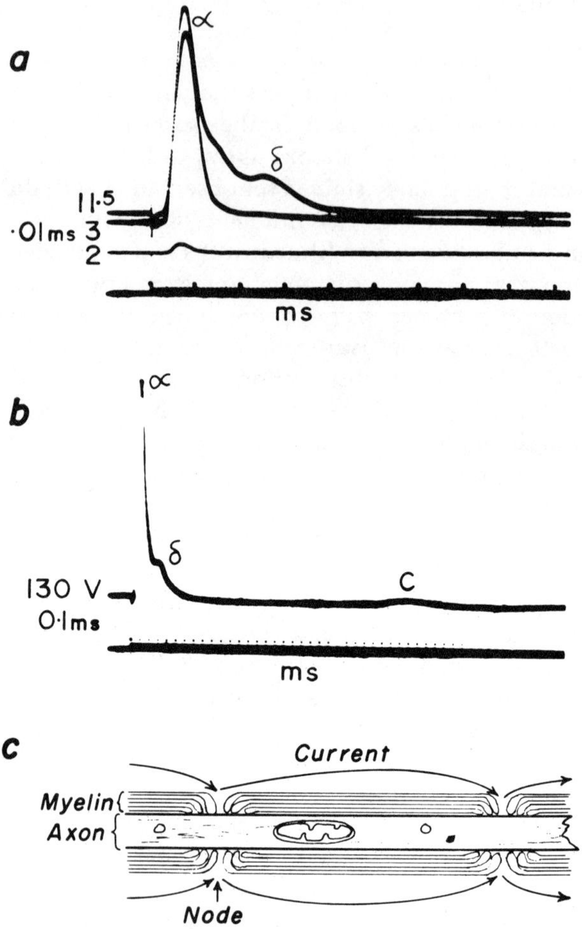

Figure 2.2. Electrical activity recorded from a nerve (maxillary nerve of a cat).

(a) A very weak stimulus of 2 volts with .01 millisecond duration activates only the most excitable—and largest—fibers, producing the small hump seen after the tiny downward deflection due to the stimulus. Increasing the stimulus to 3 volts excites most of the large fibers, as shown by the sharp *V*-shaped deflection (α). To excite the smallest myelinated fibers—the A delta (δ) group—the stimulus has to be increased to 11.5 volts. The lower line is the time signal, each notch indicating a millisecond, or 1/1000th of a second.

(b) C or myelinated fibers are activated only when the stimulus is increased over ten times (to 130 volts and to 0.1 milliseconds). The speed of the tracing has also been slowed markedly [compare the time signal with that in *(a)*] in order to include the small C deflection.

(c) Diagrammatic representation of a myelinated fiber showing the current jumping from node of Ranvier to node of Ranvier, at which points the myelin sheath is interrupted.

fine, circumferential gap at regular intervals. The exposed (uninsulated) segment of the axon is known as the node of Ranvier (Figure 2.2). The finest fibers are not wrapped in this manner but are simply embedded in long grooves in the Schwann cells. Such fibers are called *unmyelinated*, and from one or two to twenty or so axons may be contained in a Schwann cell in this manner.

Nociceptive messages are carried by the finest myelinated fibers (caliber 2 to 6 microns) and by unmyelinated fibers (diameter less than 1 micron).

HOW NERVES FUNCTION

Stimulation of nerve endings in the skin initiates a signal that runs toward the brain, slowly in unmyelinated fibers (less than 2 meters per second, or under 4.5 miles per hour) and faster (about 5 to 30 meters per second, or from about 10 to 65 miles per hour) in myelinated fibers. A consistent observation is that the finer the fiber, the slower its conduction velocity. Nociceptive messages are among the slowest travelers, whereas those from muscle flash by at velocities of up to 260 miles per hour.

The greatest difference in conduction velocities in unmyelinated and myelinated fibers is that in the former, the excitatory wave has to progress in a continuous manner along the axon, much as the burning area progresses along a fuse. In myelinated fibers, on the other hand, the impulse jumps from one bared area (node of Ranvier) to the next at the speed of electricity, a process known as *saltatory conduction* (from *saltare*, to jump). The fine features of these phenomena are known in great detail but need not concern us here.

Of interest, however, is the general process of conduction of the pain-producing signals. This is illustrated in Figure 2.2(*a*). The tracing corresponds to the greatly amplified electrical activity in an isolated sensory nerve that supplies the face. An electrical shock delivered to one end of the nerve made all the nerve fibers fire together, and the volley of impulses was recorded at the other end. Because there are groups of fibers that conduct impulses at different speeds, some arrived earlier than others, in a sequence of waves that correspond to the summed electrical activity of hundreds of similar fibers. The second wave, or A delta peak, and the long-delayed C wave are the ones that interest us, because they contain nerve fibers that relay nociceptive messages. Joseph Erlanger, Herbert Gasser, George H. Bishop, Peter Heinbecker, and James L. O'Leary of St. Louis carried out much of the pioneering work of this type in the 1930s and 1940s. The first two scientists received the Nobel Prize in Medicine and Physiology in 1944 for those studies. In brief, they were able to show that the A delta wave correlated with activity in small myelinated fibers and with sharp, stinging, pricking pain, whereas the delayed or C wave corresponded to activity in unmyelinated fibers and with dull, aching, nauseating, unbearable pain. These observations are still valid today and have provided the basis for our current understanding of pain conduction.

Conduction to Higher Centers

The sensory messages in peripheral nerves enter the dorsal or posterior part of the spinal cord over the dorsal roots, whereas motor impulses emerge from its ventral aspect via the ventral or motor roots. The cell bodies of the dorsal root nerve fibers are contained in pea-sized swellings known as *dorsal root ganglia*, within or near the bony canals in the vertebral column that provide access to the spinal cord.

THE CENTRAL NERVOUS SYSTEM AND PAIN

On reaching the spinal cord, the nerve fibers of the dorsal roots are distributed to specific sites. Those carrying nociceptive signals end shortly after entering; some of them synapse on superficially located neurons that are primarily concerned with relaying nociceptive signals, whereas others end on deeper neurons that receive a mixture of nociceptive and innocuous messages. The complexity of these central connections is such that much still remains unknown despite the application of a wide range of light and electron microscopic and neurophysiological techniques; recent summaries (Kerr and Casey, 1978; Kerr and Wilson, 1978) may be consulted for details.

It is clear that the incoming signals are not simply relayed from the spinal cord to higher centers, but that a great amount of integrative activity takes place. That is, arriving signals may be suppressed or decreased in intensity, boosted and then relayed, or subjected to any combination of such modulatory activity. This complex type of processing requires numerous local intercalated cells known as *interneurons*. To this must be added descending axons from neurons located in higher centers that exert modulatory effects either directly on the incoming fibers or by way of interneurons. The fact that these complex, integrative activities take place means that much of the business of the nervous system can be transacted at a local level, thus reducing the number of "lines," or fibers, required to relay information to the brain. In other words, the brain delegates a considerable amount of authority to lower levels and thus can attend to more important matters. Signals that are of limited or negligible importance are disposed of or filtered out locally, whereas others containing information of value are relayed to the appropriate higher centers, including that of consciousness.

However, when a noxious stimulus of sufficient intensity arrives, it is given priority; one might say it has a "hot line" at its disposal that triggers a series of important local and distant events. Locally, reflexes are set in motion that result in immediate withdrawal of the damaged area from the injurious agent. This withdrawal is entirely independent of the will, as demonstrated by the fact that it occurs both in a decapitated frog and in a paraplegic human.

What is striking about these reflexes is that they protect the organism from injury and that they are quite stereotyped. That is, a stimulus of the same intensity applied to the same spot invariably leads to the same sequence of muscular contractions—and that sequence occurs in all animals of the same species provided that circumstances are similar. This means that the circuitry in the spinal cord for such responses is quite constant and that it is genetically determined.

Another important aspect of the local circuitry is that it permits the interplay between painful and nonpainful stimuli. The commonplace observation that vigorous rubbing of a kicked shin helps to relieve the pain is explained in this manner. Of more significance is the fact that this, together with observations made by several clinical investigators such as Sir Henry Head, Otfrid Foerster, and William Noordenbos, provided the basis for the gate control theory of Melzack and Wall (1965). Practical application of this theory, as exemplified by the various electrical stimulation techniques described in Chapter 11, illustrates the value of research and theoretical concepts in the struggle against pain.

The distant events evoked in the brain are those with whose manifestations we are all familiar—the sudden involuntary pulling away of a burned finger or a hammered thumb, the cry of pain, and other more or less dramatic signs of a painful injury. For these events to occur, the message must be relayed to higher centers. This is accomplished by spinal neurons of the two types (superficial and deep) referred to earlier. They send their axons to the opposite side of the spinal cord, where they ascend for long distances, grouped together in a bundle known as the *spinothalamic tract* (because it runs directly from the spinal cord to a large, oval-shaped nucleus in the center of the brain known as the *thalamus*). The tract also provides collateral branches to a number of centers in its course to the thalamus that cannot be discussed here but are described in the reference articles.

Pain is first perceived when the nerve impulses reach the thalamic level or shortly before that. The highest level, or cerebral cortex, is not required for perception of pain, although certain parts of it play a most important role in the total experience of pain.

EMOTIONS AND PAIN

To separate pain into perceptual and emotional components is obviously artificial, since the two aspects are intimately interwoven. Despite this, such a subdivision is not entirely inappropriate and serves a number of useful purposes. Thus, the examples of human response to pain described in Chapter 1 indicated that variations in tolerance to pain are not only a matter of different sensory thresholds but are at least partly related to emotional attitudes. Futhermore, the frontal lobotomy case described in Chapter 11 provides most convincing evidence that perception of pain can be retained although emotional responses are abolished.

The areas of the brain especially involved in the elaboration of emotions are the limbic lobe and considerable extents of the frontal cortex. The limbic lobe is cerebral cortex located on the medial aspect of the brain between the hemispheres, where it follows a horseshoelike course around central structures such as the large bundle of fibers *(corpus callosum)* that joins the hemispheres. It has vast numbers of connections with deeper nuclei, and electrical stimulation of some of these centers can produce intense emotional reactions ranging from snarling, spitting, and attack to the opposite extreme of pleasurable feelings.

DESCENDING SYSTEMS THAT MODIFY PAIN

Within the past two decades, a long-held belief that the brain might be able to exert significant control over the lower centers that process sensory input has not only become a well-established reality but indeed is central to any informed discussion of pain mechanisms. Such descending systems arise form the cerebral cortex and from a number of centers at more caudal levels; they have been shown to terminate in sensory nuclei in the brain stem and spinal cord.

A particularly important system is one that originates in the periaqueductal gray substance, a rather unremarkable collection of small cells located deep in the center of the brain stem. The first evidence that this area played an important role in pain mechanisms was reported by Reynolds in 1969. He described analgesia of such magnitude resulting from electrical stimulation of the area that abdominal operations could be conducted in fully conscious rats without evoking any signs of discomfort. His findings have been confirmed by a number of investigators and applied to control of otherwise intractable pain in humans. It has been shown that a fiber tract originates in this area to reach nuclei in the lower brain stem; there it relays on other cells that send descending fibers to modulate nociceptive neurons in the spinal cord.

It should be obvious that this overview is but the bare bones of the story of how nociceptive messages arise, are conducted and modified, and reach consciousness; nevertheless, it provides an introduction and a basis for understanding some of the technical details in later chapters.

REFERENCES

CAJAL, SANTIAGO R. Y. *Histologie du Système Nerveux de l'Homme et des Vertébrés.* Maloine et Cie. Paris, 1909–1911.

HÖKFELT, T.; LJUNGDAHL, A.; ELDE, R.; NILSSON, G.; and TERENIUS, L. Immunohistochemical analysis of peptide pathways possibly related to pain and analgesia: Enkephalin and substance P. *Proc. Natl. Acad. Sci. U.S.A.* 74: 3081–3085, 1977.

KERR, F.W.L., and CASEY, K.L. Pain. *Neuroscience Res. Prog. Bulletin,* M.I.T., 16. 207 pp., 1978.

KERR, F.W.L., and WILSON, P.R. Pain. *Ann. Rev. Neuroscience* 1: 83–102, 1978.

MELZACK, R., and WALL, P.D. Pain mechanisms. A new theory. *Science* 150: 971–975, 1965.

NOORDENBOS, W. *Pain: Problems Pertaining to the Transmission of Nerve Impulses Which Give Rise to Pain.* Elsevier Publishing Company, 182 pp., Amsterdam, 1959.

PERL, E.R. Is Pain a Specific Sensation? *Journal of Psychiatric Research* 8: 273–287, 1971.

REYNOLDS, D.V. Surgery in the rat during electrical anesthesia induced by focal brain stimulation. *Science* 164: 444–445, 1969.

WILLIS, W.D., and COGGESHALL, R.E. *Sensory Mechanisms of the Spinal Cord.* Plenum Press, 485 pp., New York, 1978.

3

Headaches

Rare indeed is the person who has never had a headache, but fortunately, this most common of pains is usually of mild to moderate intensity, is brief in duration, and seldom interferes seriously with activities. Since in most instances headaches disappear spontaneously or are quickly relieved by aspirin, they tend to be regarded more as a nuisance than as a serious complaint.

Although this is true for the average headache, it is quite another matter in the case of migraines, cluster headaches, and other complex varieties of head pain. Sufferers from these severe types of headaches are often completely incapacitated for the duration of the episode. Then there are the headaches associated with life-threatening diseases such as meningitis, hemorrhages, and tumors of the brain; in these instances headache provides an invaluable warning that something is seriously wrong. Correct interpretation and prompt remedial action are of the essence if a catastrophe is to be averted.

What do we know about this common complaint? Where is the pain felt? What makes it begin to hurt? How are different types of headaches diagnosed? How does one know if one's headache is due to a brain tumor? What is the reason for a hangover headache? What has happened if you develop a sudden, violent headache? What can we do for each type of headache? Detailed answers to all these questions would require a large book, not a chapter; since this is not a book for specialists, I believe it is preferable to discuss basic ideas and give concepts of the pain-sensitive structures of the head that are involved, how they are activated in those instances in which we know the mechanism, and then to take a look at the various types of headaches, with special consideration of how they are diagnosed, what they mean, and what can be done for them.

WHERE AND WHY DOES IT HURT?

Much confusion exists about where exactly pain is felt in the head; it may come as somewhat of a surprise to know that the brain itself, the center and seat of perceptions and emotions, is insensitive to pressure, cutting, or even burning with an electric scalpel. This fact has been established on numerous occasions, in conscious patients who, for one reason or another, had to be operated on under local anesthetic injected into the skin, muscle, and other pain-sensitive structures that have to be cut to gain access to the brain. For example, operations to remove an epileptic focus in the brain often require that the patient be conscious and able to cooperate in localizing the precise portion of brain tissue that must be excised. The brain itself is not anesthetized and need not be, since, as noted above, no sensation is felt when the damaged tissue responsible for the epileptic attacks is removed; the incisions pass through normal tissue, as near as possible to the abnormal area, but no sensation whatsoever is perceived by the patient while this is transpiring.

Only the large blood vessels that enter the brain are sensitive to pain and then only for a short distance. Limited parts of the tough membrane known as the dura mater, which surrounds the brain, are also sensitive to traction and electrical stimulation. It is from these structures, then—the large arteries and the sensitive parts of the dura mater—that pain of brain tumors and other lesions inside the skull arises. They are probably not responsible to any appreciable extent for pain in the usual types of headache.

Whereas only restricted parts of the contents of the skull are sensitive to pain, structures surrounding the skull are among the most sensitive in the body. Every fraction of an inch of tissue—be it skin, muscle, blood vessels, the eye, ear, nostrils, tongue, gums, or teeth—is innervated by a profuse network of nerve fibers; as many as a thousand fibers may supply a single tooth, as in the example illustrated in Figure 4.4.

Although other structures are not quite as densely permeated with pain fibers, they still contain myriads of highly sensitive endings. Anyone who has had a severe toothache, earache, or eye injury needs no convincing on this score. It is not at all surprising, then, that the head should be such a frequent site of pain.

Other factors may be responsible for this predilection of pain for the head, but speculation enters into the reasoning to a greater degree. For example, the head is dominant with regard to the trunk and limbs and is the first part of the body that we protect when threatened with injury. This emphasizes not only our concern about being hurt but also our instinctive awareness of its vital importance for survival. Our preoccupation with the head may in part account for the frequency with which it draws our attention to something being wrong elsewhere in the body—by aching when we overindulge (hangover) or when we are upset about some problem. Speculation, yes, but with an undercurrent of plausibility that we are reluctant to reject altogether.

The two main structures in which headache pain is felt are the muscles and the blood vessels in tissues surrounding the skull. Muscular pain, not only in the head, but anywhere in the body is but poorly understood in its finer details. From a practical standpoint, a good basis for interpreting such pain is to think of what happens in the muscles of your arm when you have to hold a heavy object at arm's length for more than a few minutes. Soon a dull ache appears, which gradually builds up until the pain becomes unbearable; no matter how much one tries, finally pain and fatigue triumph, and the arm falls. All that is required is to transpose the same sequence of events from the arm muscles to neck or scalp muscles, and the development of head pain or tension-type headache is readily explained.

Pain arising from the arteries in the head is due predominantly to distension. As this happens, nerve fibers in the wall of the vessel are stretched, and the signals thus engendered are interpreted as painful when they reach the brain; the factual evidence for this statement is to be found at a later point in the discussion of the mechanisms of migraine headache.

WHAT TYPE OF HEADACHE DO YOU HAVE?

In view of the labyrinthine network of nerve fibers in the head, it is not surprising that patients describe a large variety of headaches in more or less florid terms according to intensity, location, and, particularly, the degree of incapacitation these pains cause them.

Fortunately for the diagnostician, most headaches fall into reasonably well defined categories such as tension, migraine, cluster, and so on.

On the other hand, there are others of obscure origin or those that do not fit into any neat pattern because, for example, they straddle the border line between two characteristic headache patterns. They may present considerable difficulties not only for categorization but, more important, for treatment; the more common headaches as well as some of those that are infrequent but disconcerting are now discussed.

Tension Headache

This is typically a diffuse, dull, pressure pain of moderate intensity that almost always affects both sides of the head; often the subject will say that it feels "as if a tight band were around my head." Some tension headaches may already be present on waking in the morning, persist all day, and reach their maximum at night. Whereas almost half of all people with tension headaches suffer from them every day of their lives, others may have them for only an hour or two at times of particular stress.

Mechanism. Tension headache is often considered to be the result of the stresses of modern life, but it is well to remember that past generations far back in time were subject to stresses such as starvation, plagues, and invasions by barbarians, which were no doubt just as nerve-wracking and perhaps more so than anything we have to face today.

It is not so much the stresses and conflicts of daily existence as the inability to adapt to their impact that is of critical significance in these headaches. One of the common contemporary expressions used to designate the response to stress is "uptight." Though not in the least scientific, this expression is highly descriptive of a mental and physical state. Take a few minutes to evaluate your own state of body and mind, especially if you are worried about something. Notice that even though you believe you are quite relaxed, your arm and neck muscles are actually somewhat contracted; there is a sensation of mild tightness in them. Most people can consciously relax this tension, but if a pattern of tensing up has developed, it tends to return rapidly; considerable time and effort must be invested in learning to relax if one wants to break this habit. The methods employed in biofeedback techniques are aimed specifically at this unconscious tensing of body muscles. Anxiety, irritability, and apprehension lead to contraction of muscles of the head and neck; this is not just a supposition but can be shown quite clearly by recording the electrical activity of neck and scalp muscles of people suffering from these headaches. The recording (electromyogram) shows large numbers of muscle fibers firing off in a constant irregular pattern. By comparison, when no headache is present, the electromyogram is silent or shows only intermittent activity. Also, in contrast to patients with migraine and other vascular headaches, in whom the cutaneous arteries in the area of the headache are dilated, in these people the arteries are constricted.

To treat the cause of tension, it is necessary, of course, to determine what this is; sometimes it is relatively easy to link it to some personal situation: jealousy over a wayward spouse, anxiety over unpaid bills, apprehension about real or imagined ills, worry over one's work, and so on. In other instances the causal factor is so deeply buried in the subconscious that even careful probing fails to reveal the source of tension. Something that was very important five or ten years ago is now virtually forgotten, but the disordered pattern of clenched teeth and tight muscles in the back of the neck developed into an ingrained, firmly established pattern that persists long after the responsible factor has been forgotten. The chronically tensed-up muscles do not forget—they bombard the brain with messages of tension and pain.

Treatment. Because tension headaches are of mild to moderate intensity, they usually yield promptly to aspirin. However, this is but a temporary measure—what is referred to as symptomatic relief—since it treats the symptom but not the cause.

Treatment may require considerable time, patience, and skill. If the underlying emotional problem can be identified and the victim can be helped to reason his or her way out of it, a significant step will have been taken. However, not infrequently, there are other accessory factors that contribute to maintenance of tension. True, the original source of anxiety may be recognized and relegated to the secondary place it deserves, but present sources of tension and irritation may substitute for the previous irritant.

The combination of judicious use of tranquilizers for a few months together with aspirin for the episodes of pain and, in some instances, the help of a therapist experienced in biofeedback techniques will be successful in 50 to 75 percent of headaches of this variety. When deeply entrenched emotional factors appear to be a major factor, it may be necessary to seek psychiatric help. It is important to recognize that there is no stigma attached to psychiatric therapy; much can be achieved from a few interviews with an able and sympathetic psychiatrist.

Migraine

One of the most frequent varieties of headache, migraine, can also be one of the most distressing of chronic pain syndromes. The more typical attack of migraine pain begins as a dull ache that increases gradually in intensity and then acquires a throbbing, pounding character; as the headache becomes more severe, it may lose the throbbing quality. Nausea, vomiting, and marked sensitivity to light (photophobia) are commonly associated with it. The untreated episode may last from an hour or two to a couple of days; episodes may occur as seldom as three to four times a year or as often as every two to three days.

A peculiarity of migraine is that its episodes are often heralded by signs that appear from an hour or two to twenty-four or more hours before the headache. Among these premonitory symptoms, a feeling of well-being, unusual energy, and an excellent appetite are frequent; victims soon learn to know what to expect and can often predict the time of onset of the pain.

Disturbing, but usually of no great consequence, are a variety of sensory and motor symptoms that occur just before the pain begins. Sensations of flashing lights or of a jagged, neonlike ribbon of light, which have been compared to the crenellated battlements of a medieval castle (fortification spectra), are quite common. In other instances, focal loss of vision may occur, either as an expanding black area of visual loss (scotoma) or as a progressive loss of vision to one side; this was described by one patient "as if a black curtain is being drawn across on one side in front of me, until it reaches the midline. At this time I am completely blind on one side; the loss of sight lasts for a half hour or so and then begins to recede until normal vision is restored." In other instances the victim may feel tingling or numbness on one side of the body or may be unable to speak. Sometimes they occur without a headache appearing and have been called migraine equivalents for this reason. These somewhat alarming features usually disappear within a few minutes to an hour or so, but on rare occasions they are irreversible and persist indefinitely.

Even the attack of pain may be quite uncharacteristic; the majority of attacks are confined to one side of the head, but the entire head may be involved in some cases; in others, the pain is limited to the lower half of the face (so-called lower-half neuralgia) or to the back of the neck.

The symptoms of migraine are not restricted to the head; some people have sensations of chilliness, their hands and feet may become cold and blue, and the fingers and skin feel swollen or puffy.

Migraine is no respecter of age, either, for even infants may suffer from it, and it is not uncommon for it to persist well into old age.

Women are more liable to suffer from migraine than men, in a ratio of about 60 percent to 40 percent, and the episodes have a tendency to cluster around the menstrual period. Heredity is a significant factor in more than half the cases. There are a number of factors that may precipitate a migraine attack, and victims of this disorder soon become aware of them. Eating chocolate or taking an alcoholic beverage are common causes; it has also been suggested that eating cheese can provoke an episode, but the evidence for this is not particularly convincing.

Mechanisms. There is much that remains unexplained in migraine; the most important issue of all is what starts the entire complex syndrome into motion, and the sobering answer is that we don't know. It seems likely that the primary disorder is located somewhere in the central nervous system, perhaps in the brain stem. Activation of this area or center would lead to discharge of impulses to arteries, causing them to contract or expand abnormally and thus lead to the symptoms. However, this central mechanism is a hypothesis—based on inferences but not on direct observation.

Whatever the primary mechanism may be, a good deal is known about the changes that occur in the areas in which pain is felt. Much of this information was acquired by the dedicated and talented clinical investigator Harold G. Wolf (1898–1962), who spent a lifetime trying to unravel some of the arcane problems of head pain; much of the following story was put together by him and his associates.

Most if not all of the symptoms and signs of migraine are due to dynamic phenomena involving the arteries of the head. Some of the evidence comes from the simple observation that in some patients, the temporal artery can be seen to be engorged, throbbing, and tender during an attack and that compressing it low down (i.e., just above the ear) gives considerable, though temporary, relief of pain. Furthermore, if one injects this artery with fluid under pressure, as Wolff and his colleagues did, pain is elicited. While the arteries are dilated and pulsating, however, the skin on the side of the migraine is often one to two degrees centigrade cooler than on the normal side. This indicates that the small skin vessels have contracted, and if it includes other, deeper-lying small vessels, it is possible that the restricted blood flow passing through small vessels dams up the blood and adds to distension of the arteries. That vessels within the skull also dilate during the painful episodes was shown conclusively many years ago in a patient who had a skull defect; as the pain came on, the brain could be seen to swell and bulge into the opening in the bone. However, it seems probable that the intracranial arteries do not contribute significantly to the headache or migraine, mainly because drugs of the ergot type, which abort the headaches, do so by constricting the superficial arteries but have little or no effect on the intracranial ones.

Another contributory factor to the pain may be the release of "neurokinin," a substance that has been isolated from fluid in blisters and that has been claimed to be present in tissues surrounding the abnormally dilated arteries. It is suspected but not proven that neurokinin may sensitize the pain fibers in the arterial wall.

While dilatation of the arteries appears to account satisfactorily for the pain in migraine, it does not explain the flashing lights, focal loss of vision, and sensory deficits that precede the headache. Two explanations have been proposed for these phenomena. According to one, the arteries of the brain undergo a constriction during the early phase, before the headache begins; the blood flow to localized areas of the brain and retina would be decreased enough to impair function—hence, the sensory symptoms. The other hypothesis is that a phenomenon called "spreading depression" (SD) may be responsible. SD was described almost forty years ago by the Brazilian neurophysiologist A. A. P. Leao (1942). It consists in a slowly advancing wave of suppression of the electrical activity in the cortex of the brain. In the rabbit, in particular, it is quite easily produced by a light blow to the exposed brain. The normal electroencephalographic pattern disappears, and the impairment of function spreads across adjoining cortex at a rate of about 3 mm per minute. Since the visual loss (scotoma) in migraine expands at almost exactly this rate, it has seemed reasonable to correlate this laboratory phenomenon with the clinical syndrome. However, the temporal similarities may be purely coincidental, and furthermore, why spreading depression should occur in migraine is still not explained, since no trauma is delivered to the cortex.

In addition to vascular changes in migraine, a large number of biochemical studies have been done on patients during the episodes of pain. Many of these have demonstrated abnormalities, but none of them have clarified the mechanisms yet, though they have led to more or less ingenious hypotheses that are enthusiastically espoused by their proponents and just as emphatically decried by their detractors. Evidently, little is to be gained from a discussion of the merits and shortcomings of these hypotheses.

Treatment. Since the symptoms of migraine are so varied, ranging as they do from mild episodes occurring a few times a year to severe, incapacitating attacks at intervals of a few days or even daily, treatment has to be tailored precisely to each patient's needs. Whereas a mild analgesic may be all that is needed for some migraine victims, others may require a combination of powerful drugs with psychological, dietary, and other ancillary techniques. Despite all these measures, some people have migraine that is quite refractory, bedeviling both patient and physician.

Fundamentally, methods of treatment of migraine can be grouped according to the particular aspect of the disorder at which they are aimed. Thus, avoidance of foods that are known to evoke an attack (chocolate), of alcohol, and of anxiety and stress, insofar as possible, is a first concern. The pain attack itself is treated with mild analgesics; the dilated arteries, with drugs that prevent dilatation or that cause them to contract; the emotional–psychological component, when present, by a variety of psychological techniques with or without psychotropic drugs.

Pain. Since migraine is a typically chronic complaint, narcotics are never used to control its pain in view of the strong likelihood of addiction's supervening. The mild analgesics, on the other hand, are of considerable value, and, as discussed in some detail in the chapter on drug treatment of pain (Chapter 11), none is superior to aspirin. The combination of aspirin with an ergot-type drug (see following) is one of the usual methods of treating the acute attack of pain. When it was discovered that certain drugs made the walls of arteries contract, application of this knowledge to the treatment of migraine was not long delayed.

Ergot. The source of this drug and the striking damage that it caused before its true value was recognized are worthy of a brief digression. There are strong hints that ergot poisoning has affected the human race since earliest times, but reliable reports date from the Middle Ages. Instances of fingers, toes, and, indeed, entire extremities drying up, blackening, and falling off were commonly described. Many unfortunate victims complained of severe, burning pain in the affected areas early in the course of the disease. This was the dreaded St. Anthony's fire, so-called because of the agonizing, intense pain the victims suffered and because only at the saint's shrine could the disease be alleviated and perhaps even cured. Veritable epidemics of this painful and disfiguring disorder occurred, especially in relationship to particularly wet seasons. It was only at the end of the seventeenth century that the remarkable fact was established that so innocent an act as eating rye bread was responsible.

Although the source of the disorder was at last recognized, the actual culprit remained as elusive as ever. Finally, with the introduction on a large scale of the microscope into medical and public health research, it was shown that a parasitic fungus, which was named *Claviceps purpurea,* invaded the grains of rye, and as it destroyed the kernel, it produced a hard, purplish excrescence called the *sclerotium,* which contained the poison. Subsequent chemical analysis has shown that a number of complex substances can be isolated from the sclerotium; of these, ergotamine and similar compounds are of particular value in the control of migraine headache.

These drugs have a highly selective action on arteries of the head; those to the external tissues (branches of the external carotid artery) constrict markedly under their influence, whereas the deep arteries to the brain (internal carotid system) are unaffected. A more fortunate coincidence can scarcely be imagined, for if all arteries were to constrict, serious damage to the brain might well occur; recall that the visual, sensory, and motor disturbances that occur in the prodromal (early) phase of the attack have been attributed by some to vasoconstriction. For this reason, physicians were often reluctant to give ergotamine for fear of aggravating the deficit and even making it permanent. Virtually all the research that has been done on this problem indicates, however, that such a complication from ergot is highly unlikely in view of its differential actions.

On the other hand, because ergotamine and related drugs produce strong contraction of arteries in the limbs, the risk of producing gangrene of the fingers, especially in certain very sensitive people, has to be kept in mind. Hence, the drug must be carefully adapted to individual responsiveness and cannot be used in those who are unusually susceptible. Also, it has to be remembered that ergot-type drugs produce uterine contractions and should not be used during pregnancy.

A derivative of ergot that was very successful in preventing migraine attacks is methysergide. Taken on a daily basis, approximately one-third of patients became completely pain free, and half of the remainder were much improved. Interestingly, it is of no use for treating the acute attacks. It also has a number of undesirable side effects, which in some sensitive individuals may be serious; consequently, it is used less frequently, and careful supervision is necessary. More recently, considerable success in preventing migraine attacks has been obtained with daily administration of propranolol, a drug that blocks transmission of sympathetic nerve impulses to smooth muscle of the arteries. Again, because this is a powerful drug with important effects on the heart and blood pressure, it requires medical supervision.

Although no hard and fast rules can be given for the pharmacological control of migraine, since each patient's idiosyncrasies must be allowed for, some generalizations are possible. The acute attacks should be interrupted as soon as premonitory symptoms such as unusually high spirits and energy, which the subject has learned to correlate with the episodes, appear. Ergotamine taken at this time will often forestall the migraine attack. Because nausea and vomiting often interfere with oral medication, an antiemetic drug given by injection may help the patient retain the medication. When vomiting is severe, ergotamine can be given in a suppository or by injection. Addition of aspirin to the ergotamine is also helpful in reducing pain.

In addition to ergotamine and methysergide, a considerable number of drugs of entirely different structure have been tried on migraine; frequently, enthusiastic claims for their efficacy have been followed by disappointment. At least half a dozen are being tested at this time, but it is too early to predict whether any of them will be superior to the ergot group.

From a long-term standpoint, the objectives are somewhat different. What is sought is to modify the overall picture by reducing the frequency of the attacks. Since there are a number of factors that tend to aggravate migraine, these should be identified if possible and eliminated. To a considerable degree, this involves treating the psychological basis for the syndrome.

Psychological Therapy. Stressful situations should be reduced to a minimum in these patients, who are often perfectionists and somewhat tense. Reassurance about the nature of the complaint can be of considerable help when the subject is apprehensive about the possibility of a more serious basis for it, such as a tumor. Rarely is it necessary to seek psychiatric assistance unless there are major emotional disturbances. Long-term treatment with methysergide, as already described, will further enhance the chance of obtaining significant relief.

In recent years much emphasis has been placed on biofeedback, relaxation, group therapy encounters, and transcendental meditation. Some patients appear to benefit from one or another of these modes of treatment, according to published claims. However, it is uncertain whether sustained relief can be expected.

Acupuncture has also been claimed to be effective, but no well-controlled and convincing studies have been reported; one must remain very skeptical about it for the present. Hypnosis has been used with success in almost 50 percent of cases, according to one report.

The fact that migraine in women is associated with the menstrual period has led a number of investigators to try to alleviate or suppress the episodes by manipulating the hormonal balance at that time. The results, however, have been quite disappointing.

Dietary measures may help to reduce the frequency and intensity of the attacks in some patients. Thus, careful observation by the subject may lead to the correlation of attacks with certain foods or alcoholic beverages.

To summarize, there is no "cure" for migraine, though it may become less frequent and disappear on its own over the years. However, the great majority of patients can be very significantly helped, and only rarely is migraine completely intractable to all measures.

Cluster Headaches

A particularly severe type of headache that occurs as a series of attacks separated by more or less prolonged pain-free intervals was first recognized nearly 150 years ago by a German physician named Romberg, who called it *ciliary neuralgia.* Because of its periodicity and its similarity in some ways to migraine, it was renamed *periodic migranous neuralgia* in the 1920s; more recently it was rebaptized as cluster headaches because of the grouping of attacks.

The attacks begin quite suddenly, building up to reach a maximum within five to ten minutes, and last for half an hour to two hours or so. The pain is usually intense and felt mainly deep in and around the eye. One of my patients described it as a sensation of "someone squeezing my eyeball out of its socket by pressing on it from behind with the thumb." The pain can spread quite widely to involve the forehead, upper jaw, and teeth. Associated with this, there may be tearing of the eye, stuffiness of the nose, and, occasionally, clear watery nasal secretion. The arteries of the temple on the affected side often bulge and pulsate during an attack. The skin is usually warmer than normal and may be flushed on the affected side, thus accounting for the descriptive term *red migraine,* which is still occasionally heard.

With the onset of a bout of headaches, individual episodes of pain occur one to three or more times a day and are almost always on the same side of the head; in subsequent bouts, the pain may occur on the other side, however. This pattern continues for a few weeks to a couple of months, and then, just as mysteriously as they came, they disappear, only to return several months later.

It is not uncommon for the headache to waken the patient from a deep sleep and, within minutes, for him (males are much more frequently affected than females) to be walking the floor in agony, for the pain can be so severe that some patients actually writhe on the floor and bang their heads against the wall in desperation. Unlike migraine, a family history of cluster headaches is rarely if ever obtained. The actual causative factor in cluster headache remains unknown.

What to Do? Fortunately, these headaches, because of their vasodilatory basis, usually respond well to ergotamine in the acute attacks; methysergide is also given to provide a general background of control during the period of the bout. The use of prednisolone, an anti-inflammatory steroid drug, has been advocated, and it appears to be effective.

As in most vasodilatory headaches, wine may bring on an attack during the bouts, though it has no effect during the pain-free intervals.

Headaches Due to Brain Tumor

Fear that recurrent headaches may be due to a brain tumor is often expressed by nervous, hypochondriacal, or unusually introspective people. It is not really surprising that some people should reach this conclusion, for what would be more natural or logical than for what feels like a pressure or swelling in the head to be due to something growing—a tumor?

However, brain tumors are an infrequent cause of headache, and furthermore, in the early stages of intracranial tumors, only about a third of patients are bothered by them. Thus, the likelihood of a headache's being due to a brain tumor is small. On the other hand, there is no question that brain tumors do indeed cause headaches, and by the time a diagnosis is made, more than half of such patients are afflicted with headache.

What Are the Characteristics of Brain Tumor Headaches? There is no single feature one can point to as typical of brain tumor headache, though some are suggestive. A gradual progression in frequency and intensity of headache suggests, but by no means proves, that a tumor may be responsible. The development of headaches in a person who has rarely been affected by them previously or a definite change in the pattern of headache in someone who has suffered from them quite frequently is an indication that brain tumor is a possibility.

One symptom that is particularly significant, though again far from infallible, is onset of headache with more or less abrupt movement of the head. Sometimes coughing or straining may precipitate or aggravate brain tumor headache, but far more commonly such headaches are of the benign exertional type.

Brain tumor headaches are located over the area of the tumor in about a third of the instances and are thus of little localizing value. Usually they are of mild to moderate intensity and occur in quite an irregular pattern, appearing for an hour or two on one or two days and then disappearing for perhaps a week or more, to recur in a haphazard manner.

What Is the Mechanism of Brain Tumor Headache? The explanation is relatively straightforward in most instances. As the tumor grows in size, it does one of two things: Most commonly it produces traction on pain-sensitive structures such as arteries, large veins, or certain parts of the dura mater referred to in the introductory comments in this chapter. When the tumor is located in a strategic position, it can produce sudden obstruction of the flow of spinal fluid through the ventricular cavities or around the brain. This is a much less frequent mechanism and may be given away by the fact that suddenly turning the head produces acute headache.

What to Do About Brain Tumor Headache. First of all, it is important to realize that a significant number of lesions that act like brain tumors are not cancers at all; some are benign tumors, and on occasion blood clots or other so-called mass lesions may be responsible. With modern advances in diagnosis and, in particular, with the development of computerized transaxial tomography, almost all brain tumors can be precisely localized at a very early stage and appropriate measures rapidly instituted by a neurosurgeon.

Headaches Due to Brain Hemorrhage

A headache of sudden onset and of moderate to severe intensity may be due to bleeding around the brain. If a stiff neck appears within a few minutes to an hour or two later, the possibility of hemorrhage becomes a probability, and a very serious situation may be in the making.

Although a hemorrhage can occur anywhere in or around the brain, one of the common forms is for a small bleb or aneurysm on one of the larger arteries to leak suddenly. The blood released in this manner floods into the spinal fluid that surrounds the brain, causing severe headache, and as it washes slowly down toward the spinal cord, it irritates the meninges, producing the stiff neck referred to earlier; these are called *subarachnoid hemorrhages.* When, instead of bleeding around the brain, an artery within the brain ruptures, usually as a result of high blood pressure, a blood clot forms and may act more like a tumor. Because subarachnoid hemorrhages are usually due to defects of the arterial wall, they are life threatening and must be taken care of immediately in a hospital equipped to carry out neurosurgical repair.

Meningitis

Headache, stiff neck, fever of variable degree, nausea, vomiting, and unusual sensitivity to strong light are symptoms and signs of meningitis. The headache is almost always diffuse and of considerable severity, and it is due to bacterial or virally induced inflammation in the subarachnoid space.

Coital Headache

Sudden, acute headache during sexual intercourse is a frightening experience. It is usually entirely benign but rarely can be a sign of serious intracranial damage. The most common manifestation is abrupt, intense headache occurring at or near the time of orgasm; it may last from a few minutes to hours or even a day or two. The actual mechanism remains obscure; some physicians believe it is due to the sudden rise in blood pressure that occurs during sexual excitement, but this cannot be the only explanation, since acute hypertensive episodes often occur without headache. If the headache is followed by a stiff neck or back, the possibility of a serious problem such as subarachnoid hemorrhage must be considered.

Hangover Headache

This well-known sequel to a night of merriment in which alcoholic intake exceeded prudent limits usually consists in a diffuse dull-pressure pain, often most marked in the temples and upper neck. It is markedly aggravated by sudden motion of the head, and mild cases are alleviated by aspirin. The reason for this type of headache is not known. It does not occur when blood alcohol levels are highest, but instead on the "morning after." Thus alcohol itself is not the major agent, though of course it is *the* contributing factor. Suggestions that some of the aromatic extracts in alcoholic beverages may be responsible have not been confirmed when tested. It has been proposed that dilatation of arteries and/or veins in the head may be the cause, and the fact that vasoconstrictor drugs such as ergot relieve the pain tends to support this idea.

A significant role has been attributed to psychological factors such as excitement, exertion, and, ultimately, fatigue—together with putative feelings of remose—in hangover headache. This seems to me highly unlikely, since all of the foregoing can be indulged in, even to excess, without a headache's developing, provided alcohol is not taken. Conversely, an individual can indulge heavily in alcohol while sitting quietly and undisturbed and awaken the following day with a full-blown hangover.

Apart from aspirin, adequate fluid intake, and rest in a darkened room, there is nothing more to offer for this annoying symptom. Those who are knowledgeable about it from personal experience usually have a variety of "surefire" remedies whose efficacy they are prepared to swear by.

Headache Oddities

Few people realize that eating hot dogs may produce a fairly intense, generalized, throbbing headache and that an entity called "hot-dog headache" was reported in a medical journal in 1972. The reason for this is that nitrites, which are used to give an appetizing color to sausages and certain cured meats, also produce dilatation of blood vessels. In certain particularly sensitive people, the minute amounts of nitrites contained in these foods are sufficient to trigger a headache. Monosodium glutamate, which is used in Chinese cuisine, may engender a similar headache, together with dilatation of blood vessels of the face and body in what has been rather unkindly termed "Chinese restaurant syndrome"; again, this occurs only in unusually sensitive persons.

Some normal people may develop an acute headache during sudden exertion; often nothing more than stooping, coughing, sneezing, or a sudden change in position of the head is sufficient to trigger the pain. Such head pains are commonly referred to as "benign exertional or cough headaches."

The roster of headache curiosities would not be complete if "ice cream headache" were omitted. This occurs only in a small proportion of eaters of ice cream and specifically when it makes contact with the palate. The pain is referred to the forehead, the orbit, or the temple, and in particularly susceptible individuals, it may be of considerable intensity. Dr. R. Odell Smith has suggested that it is due to a marked degree of arterial spasm at the level of the cold stimulus, which, in turn, leads to dilatation of the artery prior to the constriction; the stretching of the nerve fibers in this part of the blood vessel wall would result in pain referred to other parts of the head. Treatment for this and the other unusual headaches described requires no particular clinical acumen; it is a matter of deciding whether abstinence is better than indulgence.

REFERENCES

LANCE, J.W. *Headache. Understanding and alleviation.* New York: Charles Scribner's Sons, 1975, 230 pp.

LEAO, A.A.P. Spreading depression of activity in the cerebral cortex. *Journal of Neurophysiology* 7: 359–390, 1942.

WOLFF, H.G. *Headache and other head pain* (Revised by D. J. Dalessio). Oxford: Oxford University Press, 1975, 688 pp. s4

4

Neuralgias of the Head and Face

Not only are the head and face one of the most common sites of neuralgic pains, but some of their neuralgias are uniquely severe and, in some cases, recalcitrant to all treatment. To some extent this is not too surprising, since it is an area supplied by an extremely dense and complex system of nerves, stemming both from the spinal cord and from the brain stem.

Many different types of craniofacial neuralgias have been described, based mainly on the localization and type of pain; here, several of the more characteristic and intriguing varieties are discussed.

TRIGEMINAL NEURALGIA OR TIC DOULOUREUX

This is perhaps the most painful of all human disorders, but fortunately, it is relatively uncommon. Because of its unique features and because it can be treated with a high degree of success, it is of considerable interest. The French name for it, *tic douloureux,* is highly descriptive, since it summarizes its two most striking features—the spasmodic or sudden episodes (tic) and the essentially painful (douloureux) nature of the complaint.

This is the quintessential painful disorder, for it is marked by nothing other than sudden bursts of searing, agonizing pain, which appear and disappear for no apparent reason. There is no persistent alteration of sensation, no injury, no signs of disease of any type—just pain. The peculiarities of this odd disorder are well illustrated by the following characteristic case history.

Mike, a fifty-five-year-old salesman, felt a sudden, severe, electric-shock-like pain as he was shaving his left upper lip. The pain darted in a lightning like manner in the skin, up toward his temple (see Figure 4.1). His first thought was that his shaver had "shorted out," but he could find nothing wrong with it; after a few minutes, he completed shaving, though shaken and somewhat puzzled by the experience. The following day he happened to brush the same area of the lip with his hand, and once again, he had the same "crazy" jagged flash of excruciating pain. These episodes of pain occurred irregularly thereafter, sometimes several times a day and always as a result of light contact with that one area of his lip. Although the pain was of great intensity, it lasted for only a second or two, and after some three weeks, it disappeared as mysteriously as it had begun.

Figure 4.1. Comparison of trigeminal neuralgia *(A)* with its trigger point and the jagged, lightning-like course of pain restricted to one division of the nerve with *(B)*, the widespread distribution of dull, deep-seated, aching pain in atypical facial neuralgia.

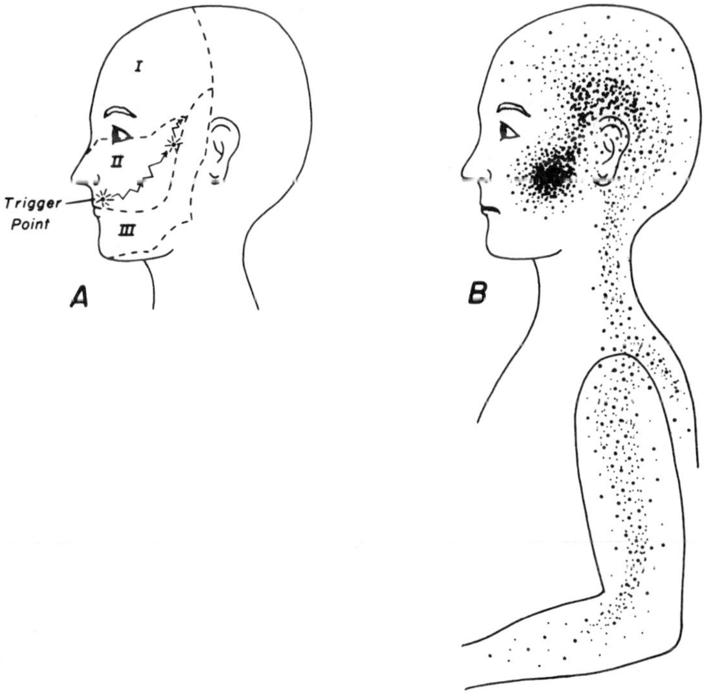

Mike was completely free of pain for a little over a year and had begun to think that he would have no further trouble when it recurred with similar characteristics and on the same side as the original attack. This time, however, the pain was triggered from his cheek near the nose, and the episodes were much more frequent; if possible, they seemed even more intense and agonizing. He noted that the pain was almost always precipitated by light touch in the one sensitive area, and by avoiding this, he was able to reduce the number of attacks; consequently, he had stopped shaving and washing that side of his face. He later was told that the sensitive area was called a "trigger point."

A friend suggested that he see an acupuncturist who was reputed to be particularly good at treating pain. It took little persuasion for him to follow this advice, and he was given a series of treatments that consisted in electrical stimulation by means of needles introduced into the back of his left hand, near the base of the thumb. After two weeks of this treatment he was no better; the severity of the attacks was so great that he had become extremely irritable and apprehensive and was unable to work. At this point he went to a physician, who referred him to a neurologist.

The latter, after a detailed examination that showed no abnormality either of his general physical condition or of the sensation in his face, told him that he had trigeminal neuralgia, or tic douloureux. He was given a drug called Tegretol (carbamazepine), to be taken three times daily, and was informed that it would be several days to a week before he could expect the pain to disappear.

This in fact was what happened, and after a month of complete relief, the dosage was gradually decreased; he remained free of pain for nearly two years, at which time the attacks recurred and were again rapidly controlled with the same medication. However, a subsequent recurrence of pain did not respond to this medication, and it became necessary to carry out an operation, as described later in this chapter.

This is a fairly representative story of the course and treatment of trigeminal neuralgia; as in all disorders, very significant variations occur in the manner in which this neuralgia affects different people. In rare instances a single attack may occur and never repeat, or the intervals between attacks may last for ten to twenty years; in a few unfortunate people, the attacks may occur at such brief intervals as to be almost continuous.

What Is Trigeminal Neuralgia?

This is a disorder of the massive nerve that provides sensation in the face and also supplies the masticatory muscles. Its name, *trigeminal,* comes from the Latin *triplets* (*tri* = + *geminus* twin) because of its three very large branches or divisions, one of which goes to the forehead and eye and the other two, to the upper and lower jaw respectively. In turn, each of these divisions has a series of smaller branches whose names need not concern us. The three large branches arise from a ganglion that lies underneath the brain and is composed of the cell bodies from which the nerve fibers arise; from the opposite side of the ganglion, the fibers that emerge form the large trunk or sensory root that runs to the brain. Figure 4.2 illustrates in a schematic fashion the position and distribution of this complex nerve.

Descriptions of patients afflicted with trigeminal neuralgia date back several hundred years; one can only imagine the terrible sufferings of those people of a bygone age whose only recourse was to pray and hope for spontaneous relief, for it is only in the past hundred years that anything effective has been devised to treat them. The intensity of the pain can best be compared to what occurs when the tooth pulp is stimulated during a dental procedure without an anesthetic.

Not only is the pain of trigeminal neuralgia of extreme intensity, but it usually occurs as a rapid sequence of electric-shock-like discharges that may last for a few seconds to a minute or two; during this time the victim is virtually incapacitated by the severity of the pain, with face contorted and hand pressed to it in an attempt to alleviate the agony. Because of its brief, repetitive, and explosive characteristics, this type of pain has been compared to the convulsions or paroxysms that occur in epilepsy; at one time it was thought that it might be a type of sensory epilepsy, and it is therefore often described as paroxysmal neuralgia to differentiate it from other common neuralgias, which, though they may have shooting pains, never have convulsive discharges. There are a number of additional striking features about paroxysmal neuralgia that set it apart from all other pains. Thus, the great majority of cases involve the trigeminal nerve, but occasionally it may affect the glossopharyngeal nerve, which supplies the area around the tonsil and the ear; extremely rare instances are recorded in which the intermedius nerve (the sensory portion of the facial nerve) or the vagus nerve has been the site of paroxysmal pain of very similar type. In each instance, these are cranial sensory nerves, but there is no properly documented record of paroxysmal neuralgia affecting the spinal sensory nerves—that is, the nerves supplying the body below the head. The number and total volume of the latter nerves are far greater than those of the cranial nerves, yet they are completely spared by this disorder!

A number of other remarkable features have been noted; for example, tic douloureux affects women more frequently than men, the right side more often than the left, and is a disorder of middle and old age. Most interestingly, in the actual episodes, after a burst or paroxysm, there is an

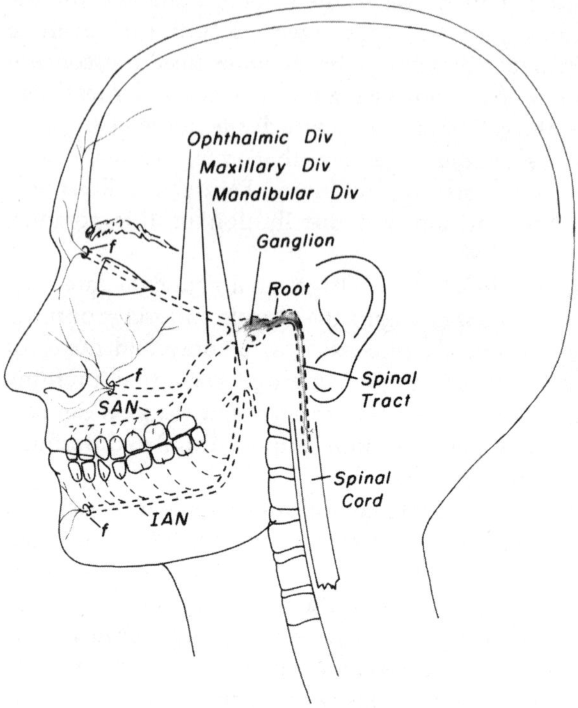

Figure 4.2. The trigeminal, main sensory nerve of the face is shown here in schematic fashion. Neurons in the ganglion send peripheral axons to form the three divisions and nerves to the face, whereas their central branches form the sensory root that enters the brain stem and descends as far as the upper spinal cord. The superior alveolar nerve (SAN) and the inferior alveolar nerve (IAN) supply the teeth. The foramina (f) are openings through which nerves emerge from the bone to reach the skin.

interval of a few minutes during which another painful paroxysm cannot be elicited. The trigger point appears to be transitorily inexcitable, as if the mechanism had exhausted itself because of the great intensity of the discharge; technically, this is referred to as the refractory period. Also quite surprising is the fact that with usual testing methods, sensation in the affected nerve is not impaired.

The reasons for all these peculiarities of paroxysmal neuralgia were completely unknown until some twenty years ago; in the past two decades, however, as a result of the development of new research techniques and intensive study, much that was mysterious has been explained, or at least some reasonable explanations have been offered. The details are very interesting to the specialist, but it is beyond the scope of this book to discuss them; for the reader whose curiosity has been piqued, references at the end of this chapter provide additional information.

The Cause of Trigeminal Neuralgia

In view of the intensity of the pain in tic douloureux, one would intuitively expect to find some more or less obvious lesion to account for the disorder. Strangely, however, when opportunities arose to study the brains and nerves of patients who had suffered from this and related paroxysmal neuralgias, nothing was found; or if lesions were found, their relationship to the pain syndrome was too nebulous to be taken seriously. As a result, a great deal of speculation developed; literally dozens of causes were suggested, ranging from softening of the brain to carious teeth; some proposals were so fanciful that one can only be astonished that the authors had the temerity to commit them to paper and that the editorial boards of the journals in which they appeared had the benignity to accept them.

For the first half of this century, the majority of specialists believed that the cause was a subtle lesion somewhere in the brain itself; they were markedly influenced in this respect by the epileptiform or paroxysmal nature of the pain, and even today, there are those who believe that this may yet be true.

However, some clues to the cause of the paroxysms had been available for years. Among these was the fact that on occasion, a small tumor or a tortuous and convoluted artery was found pressing on the sensory root of the trigeminal nerve in a patient who was being operated on to relieve the pain of tic douloureux.

Perhaps the most important observation was made by Walter E. Dandy, one of the greatest brain surgeons of all time (Figure 4.3). Chairman of the Division of Neurosurgery at Johns Hopkins Hospital in Baltimore, Dandy was not only an outstanding neurosurgeon, but he was also one of the most perceptive of clinical investigators, bringing to bear on every problem a searching intellect and a remarkable ability to identify and correlate details that others had either overlooked or regarded as inconsequential.

Dandy had developed an operation to treat trigeminal neuralgia, and in a large series of such cases, he had observed that some type of abnormal-

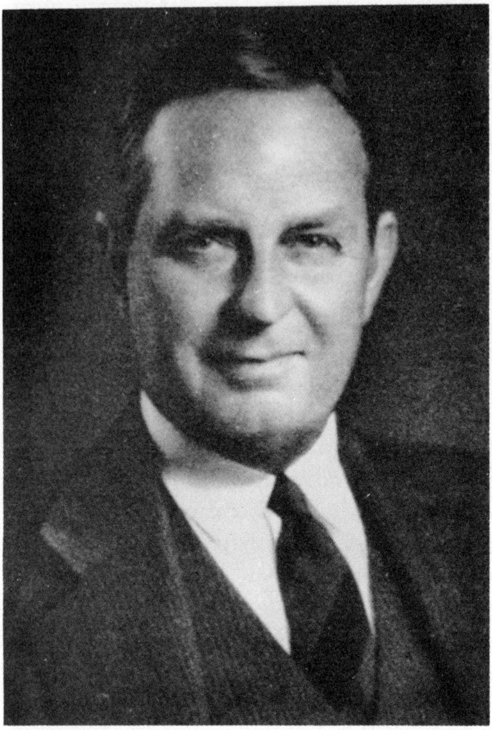

Figure 4.3. WALTER E. DANDY (1886–1946).
Born in Sedalia, Missouri, Dandy was the son of emigrés from England, where his father had been a locomotive engineer. He was graduated at the top of his class at Sedalia High School and in 1903 entered the University of Missouri. Here he came under the influence of W.C. Curtis, Professor of Zoology, who, seeing the makings of an outstanding scientist in the young man, was instrumental in channeling Dandy's activities into biological pursuits. On graduation he was offered a Rhodes Scholarship, which he declined since it required that he pursue his studies at Oxford, where there was no medical school at the time. Instead, he applied and was admitted to Johns Hopkins Medical School in 1907. Assigned to the service of William S. Halstead, Professor of Surgery and the leading American surgeon of the period, Dandy was subsequently appointed to a residency under Harvey Cushing, the foremost neurosurgeon in the world. The strong personalities of the two men led inevitably to conflict; it has been said that hostilities were precipitated during an operation when Dandy used his left hand for a purpose that Cushing disapproved of, eliciting the biting comment: "Use your right hand, Dandy, you're clumsy enough with that!"

Dandy, despite this scathing remark, was not only one of the most technically able neurosurgeons of all time, but he also possessed a scholarly and inventive turn of mind. At a time when the most talented diagnosticians were unable to localize a brain tumor correctly more than about 50 percent of the time, Dandy, while still in training (1918), introduced cerebral ventriculography, which vastly improved diagnosis and correspondingly enhanced surgical results. His contributions to the understanding of hydrocephalus, vascular abnormalities of the brain, and function of the pituitary and pineal glands, as well as the major advances he introduced in surgical technique for dealing with brain tumors, give him a preeminent position in the surgical pantheon.

Illustration from *Walter E. Dandy* (comp. by Charles E. Troland and Frank J. Otenasek), 1957. Courtesy of Charles C Thomas, Publisher, Springfield, Illinois.

ity was present at least 60 percent of the time. The most common abnormality, he found, was the presence of small veins or arterioles pressing on the sensory root; less frequently, he encountered a small tumor or some other anomaly. His astute conclusions appear to have been correct, since neurosurgeons are now having considerable success using a technique that corrects the abnormality without having to cut the nerve root; Dandy, however, used to cut part of the root to ensure pain relief rather than relying on correction of the anomaly, unless it was a tumor, which would, of course, be removed.

What to Do for Trigeminal Neuralgia

Some truly striking advances have occurred over the past twenty-five years in methods of dealing with trigeminal neuralgia. Until that time, the only effective treatment was to cut the sensory root of the nerve—a procedure that, as we shall see, brought with it a number of undesirable side effects.

Enthusiastic claims had been made over the years for literally hundreds of drugs and remedies, but in each instance, when they were critically assessed, it was invariably shown that they were quite useless. It would be unjust to suggest that this is another example of deception practiced on the public, for in the majority of instances the proponents of these "cures" genuinely believed in them.

The fact is that it is unusually difficult to evaluate any treatment for this peculiar condition because of its highly unpredictable course. Episodes of pain begin and come to an end for no apparent reason, and when medication is begun halfway through or near the end of an episode, it is only too easy to attribute the cessation of pain to the remedy when, in fact, it was the natural course of the disorder. Thus, it is necessary to treat a considerable number of patients over a period of several years before such coincidences can be ruled out in a statistically acceptable manner; this is usually difficult because tic douloureux is a relatively rare disorder.

During the past three decades, two drugs have been shown to be effective in controlling most cases of trigeminal neuralgia. These are carbamazepine and Dilantin, both of which are anticonvulsants and were originally used to treat epilepsy. Because of the marked paroxysmal features of trigeminal neuralgia, a trial of these anticonvulsant drugs seemed logical. The results have been quite in accord with that assumption; symptoms usually decrease after a day or two of treatment and disappear completely thereafter. Both drugs have some side effects, and, more significantly, they often become progressively less effective in subsequent pain episodes, at which time one or another form of surgical treatment will be required.

Surgery for Trigeminal Neuralgia

Until some twenty years ago, as noted earlier, it was necessary to transect the sensory root of the trigeminal nerve to relieve the paroxysms of pain. This operation was developed toward the end of the nineteenth century and was further refined during the first half of this century. It was the most dependable of all operations for pain, and only rarely did it fail to give complete relief. However, on one side it left the patient with a numb, dead face, with teeth that felt like wooden pegs; and half the tongue was also numb. Not only this, but loss of sensation in the eye might lead to ulceration of the cornea, and the possibility of serious infection and even loss of vision had to be considered, though these were infrequent complications. Often the jaw was paralyzed on one side, and occasionally facial paralysis occurred for a short period. However, despite all these unpleasant and even serious complications, almost every patient considered the risks and discomfort well worthwhile in order to be delivered from the excruciating pain.

One complication that was, however, extremely difficult to bear, though fortunately quite rare, was the onset of crawling, tingling, and occasionally painful sensations in the anesthetic area. This distressing syndrome is referred to as "anesthesia dolorosa"; some patients who suffered from it considered it worse than the original pain for which the operation had been done. However, since our ability to recall pain is limited or entirely lacking, it is difficult to decide which was indeed worse. One of the most distressing aspects of anesthesia dolorosa is that no treatment has been discovered for it, and it may persist for years. In summary, until the 1950s, trigeminal neuralgia could be completely relieved in almost all cases, but at a price that was sometimes heavy. Since that time a number of surgical procedures have been developed that are effective and almost completely devoid of the undesirable side effects just mentioned.

In general, these operations have consisted in efforts to produce enough injury to the trigeminal nerve or ganglion to abolish the paroxysmal discharges while preserving as much sensation in the face as possible. In this respect the operations were usually quite successful, though recurrence of pain after a few years was frequent. Today the most widely favored procedure is to introduce a specially designed needle into the trigeminal ganglion through one of the foramina (openings) in the base of the skull through which the main divisions of the nerve emerge. The tissue surrounding the needle tip is then heated by passing through it a predetermined intensity of radio-frequency current for a fixed time. This causes a coagulative lesion in the ganglion whose size can be graded by varying the time or intensity of the current and results in relatively limited or mild loss of facial sensation.

The other procedure, which was referred to earlier, was developed by Janetta (1967) and consists in displacing abnormal veins or small arteries from the root and preventing them from returning by interposing a small fragment of plastic sponge. The great attraction of this operation is that it corrects what appears to be the actual cause of the pain, and above all, it does not produce loss of sensation in the face. On the other hand, the skull must be opened (craniotomy) in order to reach the deeply placed trigeminal root. Although in skilled hands the operative morbidity and mortality should be very low, the possibility of a major complication always exists; if there is a hemorrhage or other vascular lesion or an infection, the consequences could be very serious indeed, and especially so since the disorder itself never leads to death.

ATYPICAL FACE PAIN (NEURALGIA)

Whereas the person who is unfortunate enough to be afflicted with trigeminal neuralgia will have to bear with a most painful condition for more or less brief periods until it is controlled by medication or an operation, the situation is very different for those who acquire atypical facial neuralgia. Though the pain is much less severe, we know much less about this condition and often can do very little for it.

There are few typical features about this syndrome, especially when compared with the paroxysmal neuralgias; this accounts for the descriptive term *atypical.* In fact, this disorder is so variable in its expression that it is often difficult indeed to decide which cases should be included and which excluded from it.

One of the ways in which it may manifest itself is exemplified by the story of Diane, a thirty-two-year-old mother of two who had been suffering from a toothache for a week. Her dentist found an extensive carious lesion and, after an X-ray examination, decided that it was best to extract the tooth, a left upper molar. This was done under local anesthesia without any difficulty. The toothache was immediately relieved, and after a couple of weeks she had almost forgotten about it. However, she then began to notice a deep aching feeling in and around the upper jaw, near where the extraction had been done. After waiting another week in hopes that the ache would disappear on its own, she returned to the dentist for further advice. A careful examination, including new X rays, failed to show any abnormality, so she was given a prescription for analgesic tablets. At first she believed that these gave her some relief, but after a few weeks the pain became sufficiently distressing that she felt that something more would have to be done. Her dentist again found nothing to account for this unusual complaint of pain, unusual in the sense that he had performed many extractions without ever encountering anything quite like it.

In view of the persistence of the pain and his inability to determine its cause or to alleviate it, he decided to ask for another opinion and referred her to his former teachers at the university hospital. She was duly seen and carefully examined; again nothing was found to account for her problem. She was told, however, that this might be an early manifestation of atypical face pain, since a number of patients had been seen in that clinic with similar presenting symptoms. At that time, approximately two months after the tooth extraction, the pain was deep and aching, present almost constantly, and seemed to be in the bone. During the ensuing year, a variety of analgesic medications were tried—all without success; meanwhile the pain had spread considerably and now was also felt in the temple and in and around the eye. It was always deep-seated, described as aching and bursting and, unlike that of trigeminal neuralgia, could not be elicited by touching, brushing, pressing, or rubbing the skin. It fluctuated in intensity, being mild and quite tolerable some days, but on others it would be severe, with an aching, pressurelike quality that made it almost unbearable. As a result, Diane's personality underwent a marked change; whereas previously she had been of a generally optimistic and cheerful disposition, she was now irritable and "jumpy," intolerant of her children, and had lost a considerable amount of weight.

She was then seen by a neurologist who found no abnormalities in her facial or cranial sensation and nothing of note in her general physical condition. X rays of her teeth, sinuses, head, and neck were also normal. The neurologist told her that she had "atypical facial neuralgia" and that she would have to "learn to live with it" since there was no known specific treatment; he also gave her some pills to help her anxiety and nervousness.

The pills helped her considerably, but with the passage of time the pain gradually grew worse. What was particularly disturbing to her was that it also spread progressively. Thus, four years after its onset, it extended to the back of her head and down her neck to her shoulder. At times it even spread into her arm and shoulder blade. Figure 4.1(*b*) illustrates the spread of pain in her case, which is in striking contrast to the much more severe but restricted pain of trigeminal neuralgia.

What Is Atypical Facial Neuralgia?

The preceding story summarizes a number of the features of this disorder. It affects young to middle-aged women most frequently and may remain localized in some cases or spread widely in others, as happened with Diane.

It is a deep-seated, aching, pressure pain that usually is persistent and responds poorly if at all to analgesics. Careful examination, including X rays, rarely reveals any abnormality that might account for it.

Because of the peculiar distribution of the pain, which does not conform to the known anatomical distribution of the cranial nerve roots, and because these patients are often nervous, anxious, and sometimes quite hostile, they are frequently referred to a psychiatrist with the thought that they may be overreacting to a minor discomfort or may have some kind of "imaginary pain" (i.e., "It's all in your head" or, since this is at least mostly true, "It's all in your mind," which, in this writer's opinion, is mostly untrue).

Many of the technical reasons for this statement cannot be dealt with here; they are presented in some detail in the references at the end of the chapter. However, one of the most convincing reasons for concluding that many, if not all, cases of atypical face pain are organic (i.e., genuine pain due to some abnormality and not a figment of the patient's imagination) is that occasional instances occur that are absolutely indistinguishable from the story of Diane, and that are due to a tumor or other lesion. Interestingly, removal of the tumor may result in complete disappearance of the pain.

What Is the Cause of Atypical Facial Pain?

Unfortunately, in the great majority of instances and despite the most careful, painstaking, and expert of examinations, nothing can be found. What is true is that a significant number of people with this syndrome have had a tooth or teeth extracted shortly before the onset of the pain; in some studies, as many as 60 percent had this antecedent, and it was not that a tooth had been pulled because the deep-aching pain was there prior to the extraction. Apparently the extraction is time related to the onset of atypical face pain in these instances, and the interval until the neuralgia appears is from days to a few weeks or months. Recently, it has been suggested that the cavities remaining after tooth extractions become chronically infected and cause pain; in support of this hypothesis, it is claimed that treatment with antibiotics relieves the pain in a definitive manner. However, even if this does prove to be the case, there are still many instances of atypical face pain in which no dental factor is to blame. In some cases a fracture of the facial bones or a neck injury appears to have been the precipitating factor. There remain some 20 to 50 percent of patients in whom no injury or other causal factor can be identified.

I believe that at least a proportion, and perhaps even many, of these people have neuromas on the dental nerves or on nerves in the nasal cavities or sinuses. Neuromas are mixed fibrous and nerve fiber growths that occur on nerves that have been damaged. In the case of the fine nerves to the teeth, it would be extremely difficult to demonstrate neuromas on them, not only because of their size but also because of their inaccessibility.

Whether there are people who have no organic cause for pain that they describe in terms compatible with atypical facial neuralgia and that would thus be categorized as "psychogenic" remains to be determined. I don't happen to believe it, but only future developments will settle the issue.

What to Do about Atypical Facial Neuralgia

In those few instances in which a lesion can be reasonably related to the pain, operative removal of the lesion is the rational approach and may result in a cure. However, as noted earlier, in the vast majority of instances there is no demonstrable lesion. Since medication is usually ineffective, the possibility of cutting the sensory nerves or roots supplying the affected area has often been considered and sometimes carried out. On the face of it, this is an apparently reasonable approach to the problem; what could be more natural than to cut the nerve root supplying the painful area? This procedure, as noted earlier, results in a permanent loss of sensation; the pain must surely disappear also. Alas, this much-desired result almost never occurs. To the contrary, though the pain may decrease or even disappear for a few days or a week or two, it commonly returns with all its old intensity; now the unfortunate victim has to contend not only with the pain but also with a numb face. Even worse, there may be new and unpleasant sensations in the numb area, as part of the anesthesia dolorosa described earlier. Neurosurgeons are well aware of the disconcerting fact that cutting the sensory roots does not relieve this type of pain; in the past some patients had from one to five or more roots transected in attempts to alleviate their suffering, but despite almost complete anesthesia of the face, head, and neck on the affected side, the pain persisted.

Currently there is still no satisfactory treatment for this condition. In some cases in which the pain is not too severe and in which anxiety, tension, and depression are major factors, medication such as tranquilizers, aimed at improving the emotional status, sometimes gives striking relief. However, when pain is the main problem, it is sad to have to admit that there is little to offer at present. Some of the newer procedures such as brain stimulation may turn out to be useful, but it is still too early to draw any conclusions. Acupuncture has no place in the treatment of this disorder, but hypnosis may be of some use in the less severe cases.

OTHER NEURALGIAS OF THE HEAD AND FACE

As indicated at the beginning of this chapter, there is a bewildering variety of head and face pains, many of which are difficult to classify. Whether one is a "lumper" and tries to fit as many as possible into one category—such as atypical face pain, for example—or a "splitter" who takes pride in establishing as many subvarieties of neuralgia as possible, the ultimate objective should be to try to understand the mechanisms responsible for the particular types of neuralgia and, on this basis, to devise ways of treating them. So far, efforts to determine the mechanisms of most of the neuralgias have had only limited success; in the following paragraphs, a few of these neuralgias are discussed.

Cervico–Orbital Neuralgia

This is a fairly characteristic syndrome that sometimes appears days to weeks after a neck injury or for no apparent reason; at unpredictable times, people with this disorder notice the onset of quite severe pain, usually fairly high up in the back of the neck. The pain is deep-seated and builds up in intensity over several minutes; soon deep-aching pain is also noted behind the eyeball on the same side. Associated with this there may be flushing of the face on that side and several other signs of vasomotor disturbance (stuffy nose, tearing, change in the size of the palpebral fissure). This type of neuralgia may be of great intensity in some instances and has some features in common with so-called cluster headaches, which are described in Chapter 3. It tends to become chronic and may be quite difficult to treat. Cutting the sensory roots in the upper part of the neck may relieve some of these patients, but more often there is only a temporary respite, with recurrence of the pain after a few weeks or months.

Sympathetic Neuralgias?

A number of other neuralgias have been described in which the most noteworthy feature is more or less pronounced dilatation of blood vessels, nasal stuffiness, throbbing and pounding headache, and pupillary changes; because the sympathetic nervous system controls these functions, it used to be felt that they were due to abnormal activity in the sympathetic nerve trunk that runs up the neck to the base of the skull. However, cutting the nerve, which was quite frequently done in previous years, rarely gave relief, and it is seldom done nowadays. Some of these patients respond quite well to recently developed vasoconstrictive drugs, but many are still not helped by any medication or procedure.

Postherpetic Neuralgia

Herpes zoster, more commonly known as shingles, is a painful skin disorder produced by a virus similar to that of chicken pox. The first symptom is usually a burning pain in the skin that, interestingly, affects the forehead far more frequently than the face, though both are supplied by the trigeminal nerve. This predilection of the virus for the ophthalmic division of the trigeminal nerve has never been explained. The disease may affect sensory roots in other parts of the body, particularly the thorax.

A rash of vesicles appears in the skin a few days after the pain, but occasionally before it; this lasts for about a month, during which pain may be quite severe; then in most cases, it gradually diminishes in intensity and disappears. However, in a few instances, and particularly in elderly people, the pain may persist and gradually increase in intensity. Associated with the burning and aching, there are frequently sensations of tightness and crawling, an extremely aggravating and distressing combination. In most instances the disorder appears to burn itself out, but it may take several years for this to happen.

Many operations have been tried in efforts to relieve the pain and discomfort, but only rarely have they been successful. This is probably because the pain is produced centrally—that is, in the brain itself—and cutting the nerves or roots or undercutting the skin is unlikely to modify the central disorder.

Attempts to relieve this type of pain with drugs have been, in general, almost equally unsuccessful. The development of sedative and tranquilizer drugs, however, has improved the prospect to some degree. One drug that has been relatively effective in some cases of postherpetic neuralgias is chlorprothixene; according to Nathan (1978), when given an adequate dosage, approximately one-third of patients obtain relief.

Toothache

Though not strictly a neuralgia, the pain from an inflamed tooth cavity can rival most of the severe craniofacial pains and, unlike some of the latter, can be relieved quite effectively in many instances until definitive treatment by a dentist can be obtained.

The intensity of the pain that arises from teeth is due, on one hand, to the remarkably profuse nerve supply to the tooth pulp and, on the other, to the fact that the pulp is contained in a completely rigid cavity. Figure 4.4 shows a cross section of the pulp of an incisor tooth; bundles of

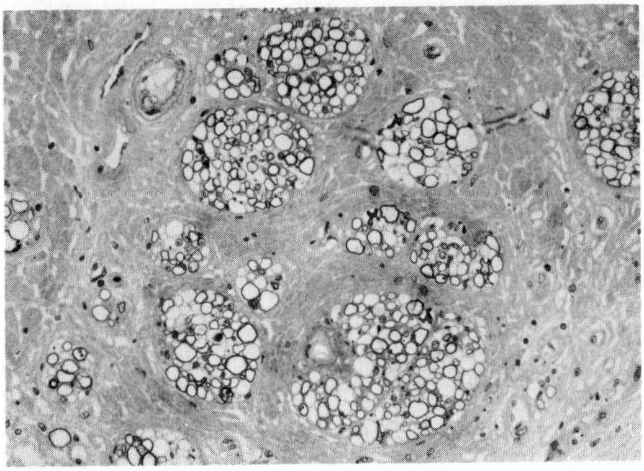

Figure 4.4. A segment of the pulp from an incisor tooth of a monkey. There are 540 myelinated nerve fibers present.

myelinated nerve fibers (the small dark circular profiles) are surrounded by loose tissue that contains scattered nerve fibers and a number of small blood vessels. In this particular tooth, there were close to 1,000 myelinated fibers, in addition to which numerous unmyelinated fibers were present but not counted. Some of the fibers are believed to regulate the caliber of the blood vessels, but the great majority are concerned with pain mechanisms. Why teeth should require such an extraordinarily rich supply of nerves is not known. Certainly they are not for sensing pressure during chewing, for example, since this sensation is provided by nerve fibers located between the tooth and its socket.

When a carious cavity reaches the pulp, this becomes inflamed; as the bacteria release toxins, blood vessels dilate, fluid accumulates, and the nerve fibers become acutely compressed with no possibility of release; therefore pain builds up rapidly. The best response to this predicament is to seek dental assistance right away, but sometimes this is not available, and aspirin or any of the analgesics are simply inadequate to control this type of pain. A very effective temporary measure is to take one of the readily available wide-spectrum antibiotics; usually within a few hours the pain will have subsided or disappeared entirely. Obviously, the condition will recur once the antibiotic effect is over, and such treatment should be regarded simply as an emergency measure.

REFERENCES

Dandy, W.E. Concerning the cause of trigeminal neuralgia. *American Journal of Surgery* 24: 447–455, 1934.

JANETTA, P. J. Arterial compression of the trigeminal nerve at the pons in patients with trigeminal neuralgia. *Journal of Neurosurgery* 26: 159–162, 1967.

KERR, F.W.L. The etiology of trigeminal neuralgia. *Archives of Neurology* 8: 15–25, 1963.

KERR, F.W.L. Craniofacial neuralgias. In *Proceedings of the Second World Congress on Pain* (Vol. 3.) (Edited by J.J. Bonica). New York: Raven Press, 1979, pp. 283–296.

NATHAN, P. Chlorprothixene (Taractan) in post-herpetic neuralgia and other severe chronic pains. *Pain* 5: 367–371, 1978.

5

Back and Neck Pain and the "Slipped Disk"

Although there are many causes of back and neck pain, one of the commoner ones is the "slipped disk"; because it causes so much suffering and incapacitation and because in most instances it can be treated effectively, it is the main topic in this chapter. It is important to emphasize that common as it is, it is responsible for only a quarter to a third of pains in those areas; the causes of the other two-thirds include tumors and kidney stones, inflammatory conditions of internal organs, and a vast number of miscellaneous factors, some of which are commented on at a later point.

HERNIATED DISKS

It has been claimed that when mankind decided to abandon the quadrupedal posture in favor of the upright, we became hostage to a whole new series of mechanical problems, centered on the spine. No doubt this new posture did result in some complications, but it is clearly not the only or perhaps even the most important factor.

Thus, quadrupeds such as the dog, and especially the dachshund, suffer from herniated disks that are so severe that compression of the spinal cord and paralysis are common. Furthermore, though estimates of people suffering from chronic low back pain in the United States range from 18 million, according to Bonica (1980), to 15 million, in Chen's statistical analyses (1979), a much greater proportion of the population is

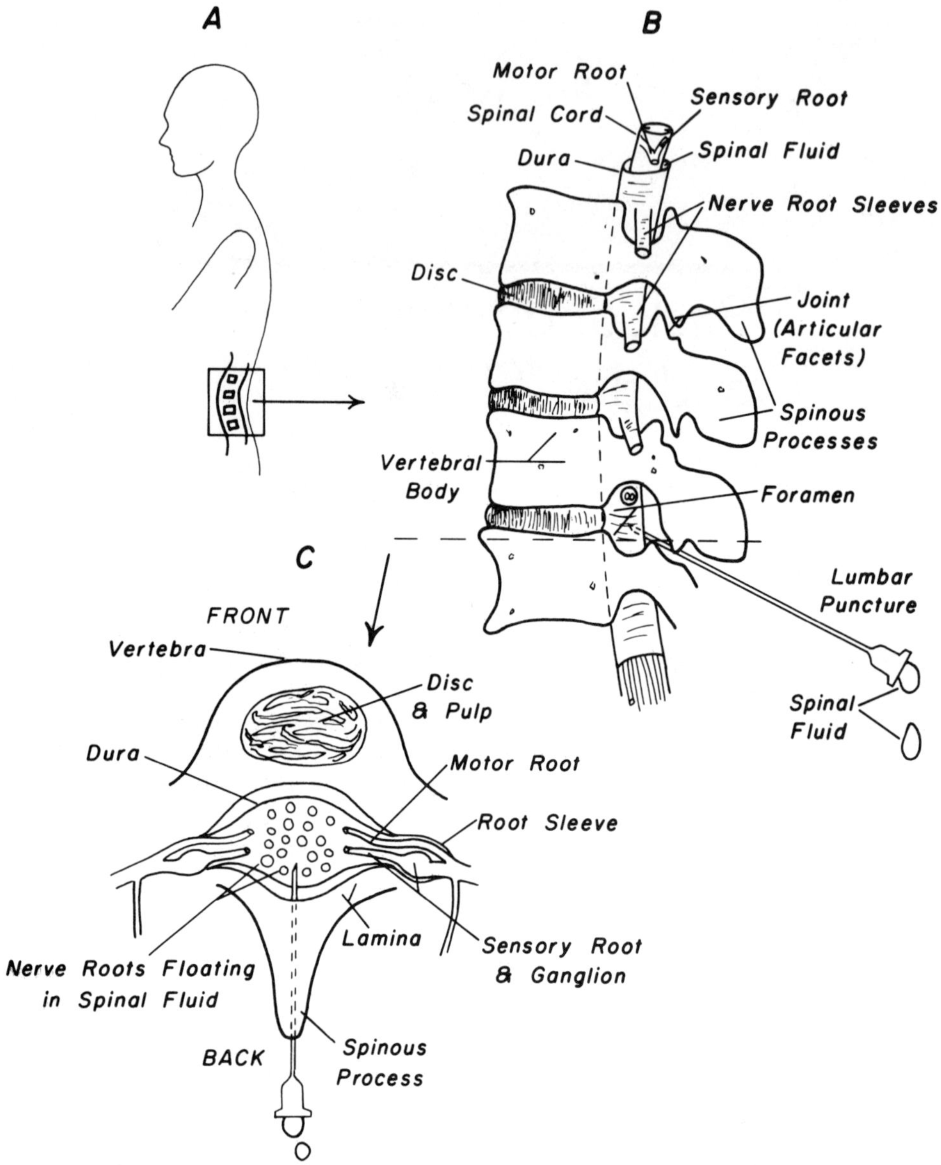

Figure 5.1. The lumbar spine and its relationships with the spinal cord and nerve roots.

(A) Orientation view.

(B) Four superimposed vertebrae; note that the spinal roots emerge through quite ample openings between the vertebrae—the intervertebral foramina. The interrupted line marks the posterior surfaces of the vertebrae, which form the anterior wall of the spinal canal. A lumbar puncture needle is shown entering between the spinous processes and piercing the dura to reach the spinal fluid: the spinal cord does not reach this point, and only nerve roots are present.

(C) A cross section through the spine according to the horizontal interrupted line in (*B;* see arrow).

spared. It is also quite striking that blacks very rarely suffer from disk herniation; in a two-year experience as a neurosurgical consultant to an 800-bed city hospital serving an entirely black population, I saw only one patient with a herniated disk who required operative treatment. Conversely, in a hospital of equivalent size with an almost entirely white patient population, a considerable part of my time was occupied with operations on herniated disks.

Thus, there are factors other than posture that predispose certain people to disk protrusion, though we do not as yet know precisely what they are; however, in the past forty years a great deal has been learned about this problem and how to treat it.

Herniated disks occur with much greater frequency in certain parts of the back than in others (lumbar and cervical), and within these areas, certain disks are far more commonly affected than others.

Low Back Pain and Herniated Disks

A common term used to describe a disk herniation is *slipped disk.* This immediately brings to mind someone suffering from more or less severe back pain, often tilted to one side, limping, or temporarily bedridden and usually guarding his or her back against any sudden movement.

The first questions we should answer about this unfortunate situation are as follows: What is a disk? How and where does it slip if, indeed, it slips at all? Why does it hurt? These questions can be answered most simply by reference to Figures 5.1 and 5.2.

Figures 5.1 (*A*) and (*B*) illustrate the relationship of the spine to the body (*A*) and of the vertebrae to the disks, nerve roots, and spinal cord (*B*). Each vertebra is separated from the one above and below it by a fibrous and pulpy cushion, the intervertebral disk. The nerve roots emerge from the spine through openings called foramina; normally there is plenty of room in this area, but a bulging disk or other abnormality can compress the nerve root and evoke intense pain, since the root can be displaced only so far before it begins to be stretched or detained by a bone edge.

Figure 5.1 (*C*) diagrams a horizontal section through a lower lumbar disk and the associated bony and nervous structures. Notice particularly that the center of the disk is composed of a pulpy substance surrounded by a ring of fibrous tissue that prevents it from being extruded backward toward the nerve roots. Many tough ligaments and muscles serve to hold the vertebrae together at the same time as they permit them a considerable degree of mobility.

During daily activity the back undergoes a variety of movements, bending forward, backward, sideways, twisting, and performing various combinations of these displacements. As a result, pressures that sometimes exceed 1,400 lbs./sq. in. are exerted on the disk, and the ligaments are

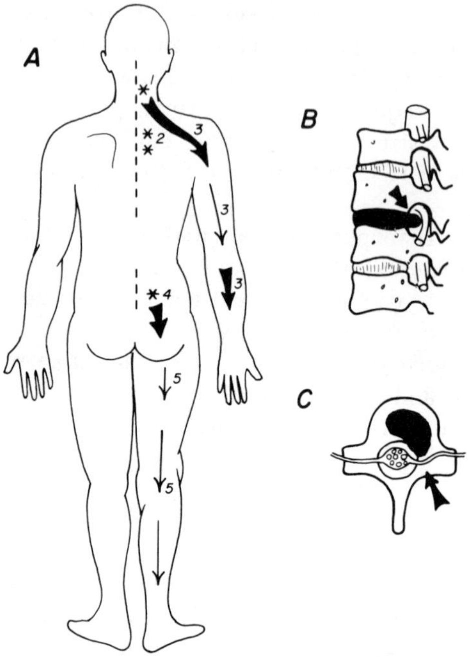

Figure 5.2. Herniated disks—the pains and some of the mechanism.

(A) In cervical disk protrusion, pain is felt in the neck *(1)* and very frequently between the spine and the inner angle of the shoulder blade at points *(2)*. It often radiates to the shoulder, arm, forearm, and hand *(3)*, producing a deep, dull, aching, sometimes unbearable pain. Lumbar disks commonly produce local *(4)* and radiating *(5)* pain, as illustrated.

(B) The protruded disk is shown in black (lateral view); it can be seen to compress and distort the nerve root—compare with those above and below it.

(C) A cross-section view of the protruded disk (black) compressing and displacing the nerve root.

correspondingly stressed. Sudden jars, as in slipping or falling with abrupt, strong, protective contractions of the powerful muscles surrounding the spine, may result in even greater transient increases in pressure on the disk. It is not surprising, therefore, if something gives way suddenly under these circumstances, as in the following instance.

A man in his thirties was working in the garden on a Saturday afternoon and bent forward to pick up a hose. There was a sudden snapping sensation in his low back, almost "as if something had popped," followed immediately by intense pain in the lower part of his back on the right side. He found that he could not straigthen up because of the pain; bent double, he hobbled inside and lay down on the couch. The pain was so bad that he felt somewhat faint and nauseated, and he noticed that it extended down into his right buttock and part way down the back of his thigh. He stayed in bed over the weekend, and the pain decreased somewhat, but when he tried to go to work on Monday, it became severe again. His doctor advised him to stay in bed for two weeks and to place a board under the mattress to prevent it from sagging. He also prescribed some analgesic tablets and a muscle relaxant. At the end of two weeks he was much improved, though he still had some of the original backache. He returned to work and several months later appeared to be back to normal. However, six months after his first attack of back pain, he tripped and fell, wrenching his back as he did so; the pain recurred immediately and was so severe that it made him cry out. This time, bed rest did not relieve the symptoms, and he felt that now there was some numbness and weakness in his right foot. Because of failure to improve, he was sent to a major hospital, where a careful examination showed that he had a foot drop—that is, he could not bend his right foot upward—and he also had a band of numbness in the skin over his big toe and part of the dorsum of his foot.

This is an unusually clear-cut case of an acutely slipped (protruded or herniated) disk. The initial snapping or popping sensation was probably due to the rupture of the ring (annulus) of fibrous tissue that surrounds the pulp (nucleus pulposus) of the disk, and attaches to the circumference of the vertebrae above and below. The cause of this situation is illustrated in Figure 5.2, where the soft center of the disk has protruded through the annulus and compressed a nerve root. When this degree of protrusion of the disk occurs, it is unlikely that it will return to its normal position; lesser degrees of protrusion, in which only a mild bulging of the disk occurs, are the ones that respond well to rest and/or manipulation of the back.

Notice particularly that the disk will have the greatest tendency to protrude when the back is bent forward. Under these circumstances not only is the posterior part of the ligament (annulus) stretched maximally, and thus most likely to tear, but pressure on the nucleus pulposus is greatest in the anterior part of the interspace and least posteriorly. In other words, the intervertebral space is wedge-shaped, compressed anteriorly, and opened posteriorly. Consequently, the nucleus will be squeezed backward against the thinned annulus. These force patterns are also of importance to an understanding of methods of prevention and treatment of protruded disks.

A more usual and less dramatic story of low back pain due to a disk is that of the patient who has had pain in the small of the back on and off for years. In these instances, the pain usually has a deep, aching quality and, because of its persistence, may become quite intolerable. It often increases abruptly with straining or coughing or bending toward the side of the pain.

Some particularly tender spots can usually be found by probing or pressing firmly with the thumb—for example, about an inch or two from the midline of the back on the painful side and in the buttock and down the back of the thigh. Though patients are often told that they have muscle spasms or nodules of fibrositis, such statements are quite misleading. Yes, muscles do go into spasm, but the spasm is virtually always due to irritation of a nerve root. When the so-called nodules of fibrositis have been biopsied and the tissue examined with a microscope, nothing has been found. The pain is particularly troublesome when one has to stand for long periods of time or sit in one of the poorly designed seats in planes and automobiles. These seats, with their recessed back support, force the low back to sag posteriorly to fill the hollow; they could not have been better designed to precipitate or aggravate low back pain.

The relatively constant discomfort in the back used to be called *lumbago*—a term that was used when ignorance was total; it means lumbar or low back pain. Intermittent "flare-ups" occur at intervals of several months or years and are often precipitated by unwise activity, such as riding horseback, traveling over rough roads in a car with poor suspension, and so on. Sometimes, after years of discomfort, the symptoms may subside, and the patient is no longer troubled by pain. It is assumed that the vertebrae may have fused spontaneously, that the disk has been absorbed, or that a fragment has been displaced to a site where it no longer presses on a nerve root.

In a number of instances the pain may be particularly severe and radiate down the back of the thigh and leg; in the past this was called *sciatica* because it followed the course of the sciatic nerve. Patients were being told what they already knew—that they had a pain down the back of the leg!

TREATMENT OF LOW BACK PAIN

Although many instances of low back pain are due either to a herniated disk, to so-called lumbar insufficiency, or to degenerative disease of the lumbar spine, there are numerous other causes of this type of pain that must be identified and treated appropriately if serious errors are to be avoided.

Thus, if an inflammation of the kidney or pelvic organs or a tumor in the spine that can cause low back pain is overlooked, for example, much valuable time may be lost by treating the symptom instead of establishing the cause and dealing with it. Therefore, a carefully established diagnosis is an indispensable prelude to treatment.

Conservative or nonsurgical treatment of low back pain due to a herniated disk takes place in two main periods. During the first or acute phase, the overall objective is to alleviate pain and avoid activities that may aggravate it. During the second or chronic phase, measures to prevent recurrence of the pain—among them, strengthening the back—are the major goals.

Treatment of the Acute Disk

During this period, pain may range from a severe, dull ache to sharp, agonizing spasms located in the low back and may radiate to the buttock and down the leg.

The cardinal rule is to rest and support the back as much as possible. The ideal position is flat on the back with a pillow under the knees if this is more comfortable, as is usually the case if a herniated disk is responsible for the pain. It is *no use* to lie on a soft, sagging mattress; this will only aggravate the condition and, in fact, is itself one of the causes of low back pain. It is necessary to use a firm mattress with as little "give" as possible. If the one you have is soft, it can be improved considerably by having a 1/2-inch plywood board placed between it and the box spring; failing this, a continuous series of rigid wooden slats placed transversely beneath the mattress will do much to correct the situation.

Then, lie on your back for as much of the time as possible for a week to ten days; sometimes complete rest for four to six weeks may be necessary. Certainly, this is a miserable situation to be in, but the alternative is worse. Change in position to lying on the side is usually necessary, since maintaining one position becomes intolerable for most people after several hours.

When getting up, avoid bending the back; roll over on your side, and have someone help you to sit upright with your legs hanging over the side of the bed. All movements should be carried out with the low back flat, straight, and rigid; twisting or flexing must be avoided insofar as possible.

Although a hot sit-down bath can be very relaxing and helpful, it is very difficult and quite risky to try this during the acute phase, and nothing can be more agonizing than to slip and twist one's back at this time! Once the pain becomes less severe and if help is available, heat applied in this manner is a useful adjunct. A safer approach during the early acute period is to apply hot packs or an electric heating pad to the low back. Occasional patients claim that they get more relief from cold compresses than hot packs.

Aspirin in a dose of two tablets repeated every four hours will help take the edge off the pain unless it is very intense, in which case a more potent analgesic may have to be prescribed by a physician. However, the use of narcotics is rarely justified and then only for a very brief period because of the risk of addiction in a situation that can become chronic. Muscle relaxant drugs may also be of some help.

Traction applied to the legs is worthless since the amount of weight that would be required to have any effect on the lumbar spine could never be tolerated. The most it does is keep the patient immobilized. In recent times some physical therapists have suspended the patient from the armpits for periods of fifteen to twenty minutes, relying on the weight of the lower body and limbs to exert traction; whether or not this is of value is uncertain as yet.

Chronic Phase

After one to several weeks of complete bed rest, in most cases the pain will either have disappeared or subsided very markedly. If it does not, then the necessity of further studies and perhaps the advisability of an operation may have to be entertained. However, most patients will be ready for a gradual, judicious return to activity; this phase includes both passive and active methods of protecting the back, as well as continued heat and massage treatments.

The cardinal principle now is to avoid flexing or twisting the back abruptly at any time. If it is necessary to pick something up off the floor, squat down with the low back rigid and flat. Better still, purchase from an orthopedic-supply shop a mechanical extension claw with which you can grasp objects on the floor without bending.

A back brace is of considerable help during this period, not because it actually holds your back up, but rather because it limits the degree of motion and protects against sudden flexion or twisting movements when one's attention is temporarily distracted.

Once the pain has subsided, the next phase of treatment is rehabilitation. Obviously, one cannot continue indefinitely with a severely limited range of motion of one's back. The objective now is gradually to increase the range of movement at the same time as strengthening the muscles surrounding the spine. This includes those directly attached to the vertebrae as well as the abdominal muscles. In instances of severe persistent low back pain, and especially if it continues to radiate down the leg, decisions about rehabilitation measures will have to be made by a specialist and supervised by a physical therapist.

In other instances in which relief has been obtained, exercises should be done on a regular daily basis and increased in number and intensity gradually to avoid undue fatigue or precipitation of pain. Exaggeration must be avoided, since it will usually set back recovery for weeks or months. Before beginning each exercise session, apply hot packs to the low back to help relax the muscles and make the exercises more comfortable.

Numerous exercise regimes have been proposed for strengthening the muscles involved in low back dynamics. One of the most widely used of these is the Williams program (1974). Because there are great individual variations in the causes and severity of back pains, in certain instances it is necessary that exercises be done under the supervision of a physician or physical therapist. Certainly, before you embark on a program of exercises for back pain, a diagnosis of cause should have been established if serious errors are to be avoided.

Manipulation of the Low Back

Since herniated disks are the result of mechanical forces, it seems reasonable to conclude that skillful manipulation of the back might reduce the protrusion and resolve the problem rapidly and efficiently. In actual fact this may occur, but there are certain risks involved that must be considered.

The most important point to remember is that one must be reasonably sure that the cause of the pain is a herniated disk and not one of the other disorders that may mimic a disk protrusion so closely that even an expert may err. Manipulation of the back in these situations may be extremely hazardous and, on rare occasions, has resulted in paraplegia (i.e., paralysis of the lower half of the body), from which there is virtually no chance of recovery.

Another factor to consider is that not all disk herniations are suitable for manipulative reduction. For example, when a fragment of disk has been extruded—that is, it lies free—unconnected to the disk space and is compressing the nerve root or, at some levels, the spinal cord, manipulation cannot possibly return the fragment to its original position and, furthermore, may result in serious and possibly irreversible damage to nerve roots or, worse, to the spinal cord if the extrusion has occurred high enough in the back. Because of these uncertainties, physicians have tended to avoid manipulative treatment for disk disease. On the other hand, osteopaths and chiropractors have been extremely active in this area and in some instances have been very successful in alleviating acute low back pain and restoring a patient to normal activities. Whether to have one's low back manipulated or not must be an individual decision.

Surgery for Lumbar Disk

When no relief is obtained with any of the conservative measures discussed and especially when loss of sensation in the skin or of strength in the limb begin to appear, the question of surgical correction is usually raised. Whether an operation for removal of the compression is advisable may be a very difficult decision to reach and will usually be made by a neurosurgeon who will weigh all the pros and cons carefully. Included in the factors leading up to this decision will be a myelogram, to give objective evidence that a disk is the source of the complaints and to establish its location. Myelography consists of introducing a radiopaque liquid into the fluid that surrounds the spinal cord and nerve roots by means of a lumbar puncture (Figure 5.1); this fluid-filled (subarachnoid) space is relatively regular and symmetrical, and anything that encroaches on it and the nerve roots in it produces a "defect" in filling that can be shown by X rays. Usually, this is a relatively simple and only mildly uncomfortable procedure; occasionally, because of difficulty in introducing the spinal needle, it can be quite disagreeable and painful. If the myelogram confirms the diagnosis, removal of the herniated disk will be the next step.

To remove a protruded disk, the surgeon has to resect a part of the bony arch that overlies the root; this bone is called the lamina [see Figures 5.1(*C*) and 5.2(*C*)]; since only part of one side of it is removed, the operation is called a partial hemilaminectomy. Following this, the nerve root is carefull displaced, and the protruded disk is gently teased out. This operation should only be performed by surgeons with special training, since it is not simple, and complications of a serious nature can occur on rare occasions.

When the patient awakens from the anesthetic, it is not uncommon for the buttock and leg pain to have disappeared completely; however, some patients will have a variable degree of pain from the incision, and occasionally muscle spasms may occur for several days. After two to four days, there will usually be very little discomfort, and carefully controlled ambulation (walking) can begin twenty-four to forty-eight hours postoperatively.

The following are some commonly asked questions about surgery for lumbar disks.

Q: If the disk is removed, what is it replaced by?

A: Usually nothing is replaced; the degenerated disk was performing no useful function, and in its absence, the vertebrae usually adapt to each other without trouble. In some cases the vertebrae on either side of the missing disk may actually fuse together.

Q: Is one likely to be paralyzed as a result of a lumbar disk or by surgery for it?

A: Because these disks are almost always in the lower lumbar spine and thus below the tip of the spinal cord, the answer is no. However, once in many operations a localized paralysis or weakness of the muscles may occur; sometimes this is only a temporary aggravation of weakness that was already present. At other times it may be a result of damage to a root that was particularly difficult to decompress. The likelihood of recovery from such weakness is uncertain, and permanent weakness may remain.

Q: Is impotence or bladder weakness likely to occur after surgery?

A: Although the nerves to the genital organs and bladder do pass by the disk, they are usually too far away to be affected. However, as noted at other points in this chapter, there is very little that can be answered with 100 percent certainty in medicine; nevertheless, such complications are quite unlikely. Difficulty in emptying the bladder and bowels is common for a few days postoperatively, but except for very rare instances, it disappears without leaving any deficit. Occasionally, a very large extruded disk may compress the nerves to the bladder and produce difficulty or inability in voiding.

Q: Is it necessary to perform a fusion of the vertebrae to strengthen the back or prevent a recurrence?

A: Though some surgeons still perform fusions at the end of laminectomies, the majority do not, other than in a few special circumstances. In general the answer is no.

Q: Will I require a back brace permanently after surgery?

A: With successful surgery, a back brace will rarely if ever be needed.

Q: What are the chances of having a successful result from an operation?

A: If it is the first operation for the disk, and it is done by a highly qualified surgeon, there is a better than 80 percent chance of having a good to very good result.

Q: What is a very good result?

A: This may range from no further pain at all to only minor, intermittent low back discomfort. Return to full normal activity can be expected.

NECK PAIN AND CERVICAL DISKS

Like low back pain, neck pain due to a disk is both common and exceedingly unpleasant. The onset is quite similar to lumbar pain in that pain is felt near the midline and is often precipitated by strain or sudden, more or less violent movement; on the other hand, a bout of coughing or some even more trivial movement is enough to produce it; a commonly used term to describe this type of pain is *wry neck*.

A typical onset may occur when backing a car out of a parking place; the head is acutely turned to one side, and a sudden sharp pain is felt, usually low in the neck. The pain may increase in severity and become of such intensity that the slightest movement or jarring results in waves of pain of such intensity as to produce nausea. As in the case of low back pain, it is usual for the patient to have episodes of pain lasting for a few days to weeks interspersed with pain-free periods of months or even years.

During the individual bouts of pain, in addition to the aching and occasional stabbing pain in the neck, it is very common to have quite intense aching pain in the back along the upper and inner margin of the shoulder blade on the same side; the pain is very localized and covers an area not much bigger than the tip of one's finger; for each intervertebral level, there is a specific level where pain is felt (Figure 5.2). Pain may radiate down the arm on one side; it is of a dull aching type and seems to be deep in the muscle or in the bone; it may be felt in the back of the arm, the forearm, the wrist, and occasionally in the hand. Surprisingly, pain is often felt in the chest as if it were in the breastbone (sternum) or in the ribs, near it. It is not at all uncommon for these deep, aching pains, especially when localized in the arm or hand, to be misdiagnosed as rheumatism or arthritis; a more or less prompt response to neck traction, however (see below), resolves any doubts about the cause! Some people may also develop headaches as a result of spasm of neck muscles resulting from a herniated cervical disk.

When the disk protrusion is pronounced or a fragment of disk is actually extruded and lies wedged against a nerve root, in addition to pain there may be numbness in the skin and weakness of the muscles supplied by the involved root.

Treatment of Cervical Disk Pain

Mild episodes of neck pain due most probably to slight protrusion of a disk will usually subside on their own in a few days to a week or so. The natural tendency of the muscles to contract and keep the neck relatively immobilized is often enough to alleviate pain and prevent further progression. However, this is a period when a person is "at risk," since any sudden movement of the head may result in marked or even serious aggravation of the condition; abrupt increase in pain may be due to further protrusion of the disk, whereas serious progression is sometimes the result of actual extrusion of a disk fragment.

Manipulation or "adjustments" of the neck carry a potentially serious risk, since the spinal cord may be damaged directly by a large disk fragment that is displaced against it by the manipulation. Furthermore, at least twenty-six reported cases of infarction (stroke) affecting the posterior brain as a direct result of manipulation of the neck have been collected recently by Krueger and Okazaki (1980), who have reported an additional nine cases of this complication, one of whom, a twenty-five-year-old man, died.

It is always difficult to predict what will happen with an acute episode of neck pain, but the safest conduct is to take preventive measures right away. The simplest of these is to wear a "Thomas collar"; this is a relatively rigid collar some three inches high, made usually of plastic or of heavy cardboard with a foam rubber or other protective covering that fits snugly around the neck and limits head movement in any direction. This should be worn constantly during the day and in some instances round the clock if pain is particularly severe.

Usually it can be removed at night and replaced with a rolled pillow placed under the neck so that when lying on one's back, the head is slightly extended, as shown in Figure 5.3(*A*). Additional relief may be obtained by raising both arms up beside the head for periods of five to ten minutes. It is not uncommon to awake after a night's sleep in this position and find that the neck pain has dissapeared.

A simple maneuver that is helpful in relieving mild to moderate neck pain is to raise the head as much as possible—when driving or walking, for example. Perhaps the best way to describe this is that one stretches one's neck upward as if trying to look over a high fence. Almost immediate alleviation of neck pain and often of the deep aching pain in between the shoulder blades, in the arm, forearm, wrist, or hand often occurs when this

Figure 5.3. Conservative treatment of cervical disk protrusions.
(A) A rolled pillow under the neck to produce extension when lying in bed.
(B) Cervical traction by means of a canvas halter; the head can be in the neutral position, as illustrated, or extended; the separation of the vertebrae helps the disk to return to its normal location.

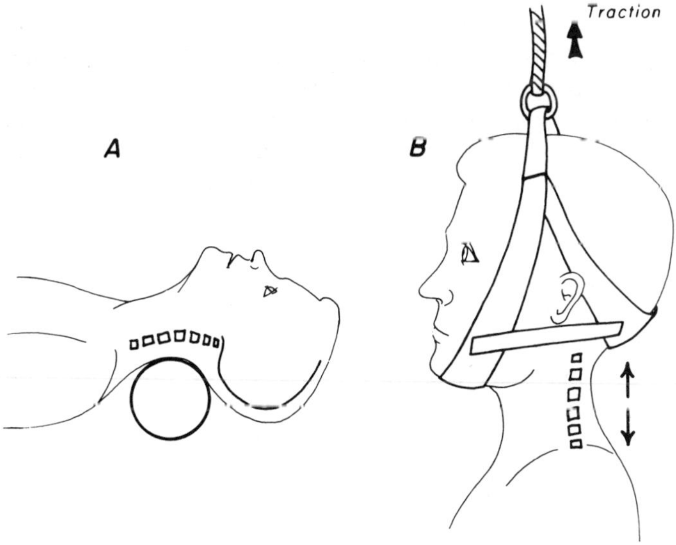

maneuver is done correctly. Sometimes bending the head backward for several minutes will help ease pain.

When neck pain is more severe or does not respond to these maneuvers, traction applied to the head will often provide rapid and striking relief. Because in a small percentage of cases, traction can aggravate neck pain and even produce serious damage to the nerve roots or spinal cord, medical advice and supervision should be sought; as noted previously, on rare occasions a tumor or other disorder involving the nerve roots or spinal cord may produce symptoms that are difficult to distinguish from those resulting from a protruded disk.

Traction is applied to the head by means of a canvas halter, as illustrated in Figure 5.3(*B*). Here the subject is in a sitting position with a cord from the halter passing up and over a pulley attached to a secure overhead beam. The degree of traction can be varied from a few pounds to thirty or forty or more; the decision as to how much is the responsibility of the physician.

The position of the head is important; it should be either neutral or slightly extended (i.e., bent backward); there is some controversy over this point, since a number of physical therapists advise a flexed position of the head (bent forward about 20°) during traction because this tends to open the interspace posteriorly and theoretically helps to return the protruded disk to its normal position. However, the mechanics of the interspace, as discussed earlier in this chapter, are such that flexing the head tends to squeeze the intervertebral disk backward, whereas extending it—especially when small nodding and turning movements are made from side to side while in traction—is much more likely to be effective. In my own experience a slightly extended position of the head produces more rapid relief. The subject should try to relax all neck and shoulder muscles and, after some three to four minutes, should begin gently to extend and flex the head, alternating this with slight rotation movements to the right and left. I have not come across any description in the literature of associating movement of the head with traction in this manner but have found that it accelerates recovery quite significantly. The objective is to "jockey" the protruded disk back into position; though not always successful, it frequently achieves its objective.

Traction should be applied for periods of five to ten minutes two to three times daily if possible. When traction is to be applied in the supine position, in bed, it is necessary to raise the head of the bed to provide countertraction from the body. In all instances, traction should be applied gradually until the full intensity is reached; particularly important, it should be decreased slowly at the end of the session. When a Thomas collar is being worn, it should be replaced immediately after the traction session is over.

By following the foregoing schedule, most cases of neck pain due to a protruded disk will be relieved after three or four days; occasionally treatment will have to be continued for a week or two. If pain continues after this length of time, and especially if loss of sensation in the skin or muscle weakness is present, it may be necessary to consider an operation for removal of the disk and decompression of the affected nerve root; however, in the great majority of cases of disk pain, operation can be avoided.

Operative results in competent hands are very satisfactory in cervical disk protrusion, with permanent relief in about 90 percent of cases. Whether the disk will be removed from a posterior or anterior approach is a matter the surgeon must decide. Opinions remain divided as to the merits of each approach.

Traction leading to relief of neck pain should be supplemented by preventive measures aimed at avoiding recurrence. Anyone who has had an episode of acute neck pain, especially if it has radiated into the arm or between the shoulder blades, is aware of being more susceptible to it than the average person; by following the simple rules summarized next, one can markedly reduce the likelihood of a recurrence.

1. Avoid sitting with your head bent forward—that is, with chin on or near the chest.
2. Never go to sleep with your head pressed against the headboard; that is, avoid vertical pressure on your head.
3. As soon as you feel neck pain or any pain that you have come to associate with your neck, stop what you are doing, stretch your neck up as much as possible, and bend it slightly backward.
4. If the symptoms persist, use a Thomas collar for a few days; traction twice daily for several days will usually relieve the problem.
5. If at any time you have a sudden severe episode of neck pain, and especially if it is accompanied by radiation down your arm, see a physician; you may have a ruptured disk with an extruded fragment. When in doubt, seek medical advice.

It is questionable whether neck exercises are of value in avoiding recurrence of pain due to cervical disk.

While the great majority of neck pains respond to the preceding treatment and variants thereof, there are still a number of patients who have chronic neck and/or arm pain that is not relieved by any of these measures. The pain is due to compression of nerve roots by bony protrusions into the intervertebral foramen in some patients with severe arthritis of the neck; in others, to chronic inflammatory changes around nerve roots; but in some of these situations the cause of pain remains obscure, and treatment is relatively unsatisfactory.

FAILED LOW BACK SYNDROME

Regardless of how skilled a surgeon is, a certain percentage of patients who have what may appear to be a lumbar disk syndrome respond poorly or not at all to being operated on. In attempts to improve on this situation, a patient may have surgery on a number of occasions, and instances of five, six, or more operations are not uncommon. Unfortunately, with each succeeding operation, the prospect of relief becomes progressively more remote; frequently such patients become chronic cripples.

The reasons for these failures are complex and often unknown. Sometimes a chronic low-grade inflammatory process known as arachnoiditis appears to be responsible, and in others scarring around the nerve roots may be at fault. More often than not, it is difficult or impossible to determine the cause of the problem, and in a number of instances psychogenic problems play an important role.

Electronic stimulators have been used with some success, but after initially favorable results, failure appears to be the rule. At this time, there is relatively little that can be done for most of these patients, though sporadic, highly successful results with any one of a variety of treatments are reported.

One seemingly logical way to relieve the pain in these unfortunate situations is to sever the sensory root (dorsal rhizotomy). This approach was tried over thirty years ago for failed disk operations, but the results were quite disappointing, and most surgeons have therefore been reluctant to advise this operation. Another procedure that was first reported some five years ago is to remove the dorsal root ganglion [see Figure 5.1(*C*)].This operation (ganglionectomy) is too recent for any definitive opinion to be expressed. However, Hosobuchi (1980) has now reported on three patients who had undergone dorsal rhizotomy for severe chest pain without any relief. Subsequently, dorsal ganglionectomy gave two patients complete relief of pain up to the time of the report (three years); one patient had significant improvement. The obvious conclusion was that the ventral or motor roots contained fibers whose cell bodies were in the dorsal root ganglion and had thus had escaped transection during the initial operation.

The operation is currently being evaluated in patients with failed disk procedures and in selected instances may well prove to be a significant advance in therapy.

OTHER CAUSES OF LOW BACK PAIN

When disks, arthritis, congenital malformations, mechanical imbalances such as a shorter leg, osteoporosis of the spine, tumors and inflammations of the vertebrae or of the pelvic organs have all been ruled out, there remains a substantial group of people in whom no causal factor can be identified but who continue to complain of low back pain. Many knowledgeable physicians consider that such complaints are basically psychogenic and that the pains will not be relieved until the patients' emotional problems have been resolved.

In conclusion, pain problems are often difficult to diagnose and treat, but some low back pain problems are often in a class all by themselves in terms of complexity and intractability.

REFERENCES

BONICA, J.J. Conclusion in Pain, *Res. Publ. A.R.N.M.D.* Vol. 58: 381–384. New York: Raven Press, 1980.

CHEN, T.C. In "Panel in Pain" National Advisory, Neurologic and Communicative Disorders and Stroke Council, Department of Health, Education and Welfare, Washington, D.C., 1979.

KRUEGER, B.R., and OKAZAKI, H. Vertebral-basilar distribution infarction following chiropractic cervical manipulation. *Mayo Clinic Proceedings.* 55: 322–332, 1980.

SPANGFORT, E.V. The lumbar disk herniation. *Acta Orthop. Scand. Suppl.* 142: 1–95, 1972.

WILLIAMS, P.C. *Low back and neck pain.* Springfield, Ill.: Charles C. Thomas, 1974, 78 pp.

6

Cancer and Pain

Four hundred thousand deaths every year in the United States from cancer!—a grim statistic, indeed, but conveying nothing of the human anguish and pain this relentless disease inflicts on its victims. More than half of them, or approximately a quarter of a million people, will be suffering from chronic pain at the time of death (Bonica 1980). In some, pain appears only toward the end, but in others it is the presenting symptom, lasting anywhere from months to a year or two; its intensity ranges from mild to intolerable.

No wonder, then, that it is one of the most feared of all diseases, for not only does it cripple, disfigure, and kill, but it often does so slowly and painfully. Yet much of the suffering it causes could be relieved and often abolished with means that are already at hand. That full advantage is not taken of these measures is due mainly to lack of understanding of the problem. What is needed is a much more effective approach that encompasses not only technical expertise in the management of pain but also humanitarian and compassionate care programs for these unfortunate patients.

WHY DOES CANCER CAUSE PAIN?

The most obvious and perhaps most common mechanism of pain in cancer is pressure and distortion of sensitive structures. Since cancer consists in the uncontrolled growth of cells, they soon form a mass or tumor. When much room is available in a body cavity—such as the abdomen, for example—a tumor may reach a considerable size before pain is felt; the opposite occurs when a tumor happens to grow in a confined area. For example, tumors growing in bones produce pain quite early in their course, either because they are confined within a bony cavity (marrow or sinus) or because they stretch and distort the periosteum. The latter, a fine fibrous membrane that envelops the surface of bones, is richly supplied with pain fibers. Abrupt aggravation of pain may also occur when a tumor has destroyed the bone structure to the point where it collapses; this is known as a pathological fracture.

In other instances, tumors may infiltrate and stretch nerves or the nerve plexuses that supply the limbs. Pain may be localized to the plexus or may radiate out along the limb in a pattern corresponding to the nerves involved; it is usually dull and aching or burning in quality.

The preceding examples of cancer pain are all due to mechanical processes—compression, stretching, distortion of nerve fibers—but this is not necessarily the only mechanism. Obstruction of blood and lymph vessel, blockage of viscera such as the bowel or ureter, and the possibility that tumors may secrete or cause the release of toxic, pain-producing substances also have to be considered. And, when radiotherapy has been given, scar tissue may develop and lead to the delayed onset of pain as nerve fibers are trapped and compressed.

Relief of Pain in Cancer

Anything that will make a tumor regress or involute will, in all probability, reduce or abolish the pain it has been causing. Chemotherapy is one means of accomplishing this objective, but as yet it is effective only in a small proportion of tumors; furthermore, the solid tumors—that is, those that form masses and are most commonly responsible for pain—are particularly resistant to chemotherapy.

Radiotherapy may be very effective in certain tumors, and as they involute under the influence of radiation, pain decreases. However, as already noted, postradiation scarring can cause chronic pain, which is then difficult to control.

Drug treatment of the pain itself consists in using the weak analgesics such as aspirin when pain is mild. When aspirin is no longer effective, the stronger analgesics are employed. As discussed in Chapter 10, a number of new, powerful synthetic analgesics are currently being introduced (see page 135), some of which are claimed by their developers to be as potent as morphine and, moreover, are said to lack the addictive properties of narcotics. In patients with pain due to cancer, however, addiction is a nonissue, since the overriding concern is to suppress the pain; whatever dose of morphine is necessary to achieve the desired effect should be used as frequently as needed to provide comfort. Beginning with the lowest dose of morphine that relieves the pain, the dosage is increased gradually to keep abreast of increments in pain, as the cancer increases in size, and to overcome the tolerance (see Chapter 10) that develops.

It is absolutely useless to prescribe the standard dose of 10 mg of morphine every four hours if it does not give adequate respite from pain. And if it is initially effective, within a few days the rapid increase in tolerance to narcotics that occurs with repeated administration will already neutralize most of its action. Yet this unimaginative treatment of cancer pain is not infrequent, sometimes because of a lack of understanding of drug action and occasionally from a callous disregard for suffering.

Another relatively simple method of alleviating cancer pain that is enjoying a considerable measure of popularity at this time is the so-called Brompton cocktail, first prescribed for cancer pain by the English surgeon Snow at the end of the nineteenth century. The mixture contains morphine, cocaine, alcohol, syrup, and chloroform water; earlier formulas contained gin and honey, according to Twycross (1979). In efforts to improve its efficacy, morphine has been replaced with heroin (diacetyl morphine) but without significant improvement in results (Twycross). If to this is added the extremely grave abuse potential of heroin, and the much readier general access to this dangerous drug that would occur if current restrictions were relaxed to permit its use, it seems obvious that the ban should not be lifted; there is, of course, no reason to be concerned about addiction in a patient with pain due to cancer.

When pain cannot be adequately controlled by narcotics, when they are poorly tolerated, or when they are producing marked confusion with inadequate pain relief, there are a number of other techniques of pain control that can and should be used. These include nerve blocks and neurosurgical procedures such as cordotomy, brain stimulation, and hypophysectomy (see Chapter 11). In skillful hands, nerve blocks can be of great value in controlling pain, as pointed out by Bonica (1980), Gerbershagen (1979), and many others. A nerve block consists in the injection of either a local anesthetic or an agent such as alcohol or phenol, which will interrupt the peripheral pain pathway by causing degeneration of the nerve fibers supplying the area invaded by the tumor.

In most instances one or more nerve blocks with local anesthesia will be done. This serves a double purpose since, first of all, it allows the patient to experience what the sensation of numbness will be like if this is to occur, and how well he or she is likely to tolerate it, before proceeding to the more permanent destructive blockade with alcohol, for example. The other advantage is that it helps to determine whether the pain is likely to be satisfactorily controlled by a "permanent" block. Interestingly, it is not uncommon to obtain pain relief lasting for days and sometimes for weeks after two or more injections of local anesthetic. In successful instances, pain can be suppressed in this manner for periods of four to six months (Gerbershagen).

Another method of control of cancer pain that has been used with considerable success is injection of a dilute solution of phenol into the spinal fluid at the level of the sensory nerve roots that are carrying the pain input from the tumor area.

Neurosurgical procedures for the relief of cancer pain can be of considerable value in carefully selected instances. Their advantages and shortcomings are referred to in Chapter 11.

From the preceding summary of methods of control of pain from cancer, the reader may conclude that any pain of this origin can be relieved by one or more of these techniques. Unfortunately, this is not always the case; there are still a significant number of patients whose pain cannot be completely controlled, and further research, both on drugs and on other methods of modifying the nerve pathways concerned with pain, is still very much needed.

Intermittently over the years, hypnosis has been used to relieve pain from cancer. As noted in Chapter 13, one of the first reported instances of painless surgery under hypnotic suggestion was carried out on a patient who had previously been relieved of cancer pain with this technique.

In recent years hypnosis has been used successfully for the relief of both anxiety and pain due to cancer in a number of instances; the following case history, representative of results that can be achieved in this way, is reproduced by kind permission of Dr. Joseph Barber of the U.C.L.A. Pain Unit.

> Mark, a 42-year-old pharmaceutical company executive, was diagnosed as having testicular cancer. He had intense pain in his pelvic area and was fearful of becoming addicted to the narcotics used to treat pain. He was unable to accept his physician's report that his cancer was progressing rapidly and that his illness could not be cured. He insisted that there must be a drug to help him and began to make plans to travel to Mexico for Laetrile treatment.
>
> He would not follow instructions and tried to plan his own treatment; he was depressed, showed inappropriate denial of illness and made unrealistic plans for marriage despite the unfavorable prognosis.
>
> Hypnosis was prescribed and after some initial resistance, he began to relax and to accept instructions of the hospital staff. His anxiety decreased and he was taught to induce self-hypnosis to help control his pelvic pain. Pain control was maintained without narcotics until two weeks prior to his death. Even then, narcotic dosages were minimal.

THE HOSPICE CONCEPT

The first modern institution dedicated exclusively to the care of people with chronic long-term illness, and in particular to that of patients with advanced cancer, was St. Christopher's Hospice at Sydenham, England. Since its inception in 1967, a number of units patterned along similar lines have been developed both in Britain and in other countries. Examples are the Continuing Care Units in Britain; the Home Care Team in New Haven, Connecticut; the Symptom Control Team at St. Luke's Hospital, New York; and the Palliative Care Unit and Service at the Royal Victoria Hospital in Montreal, Canada.

The objective of these centers is to provide a combination of skilled medical and nursing care, with special emphasis on control of pain, together with a warm and receptive community environment in which the patient can feel secure and cared for as a human being. By means of a home care program, patients are able to return to their homes for variable periods of time and to be readmitted at the time of their choice for additional care when and if the family environment cannot cope.

From several case histories quoted by Dr. Cicely Saunders (1979) of St. Christopher's Hospice, I have selected two as representatives of what can be accomplished.

A woman with a one-year history of intractable pain due to cancer of the pancreas was admitted to St. Christopher's Hospice for the last eleven weeks of her life. A friend of hers wrote the following letter to Doctor Saunders:

> It was nothing short of a miracle. When I last visited her in a previous hospital she was like a demented animal—consumed with pain, incoherent of speech, and quite vicious. I was very frightened, not knowing how to cope, and felt unable to face another visit. Words cannot describe my reaction when I saw her in St. Christopher's—restored to the dignity of a calm, rational human being again. . . . From then on I was able to remain with her for hours at a time, instead of minutes, holding conversation and discussing things of interest dear to her heart. . . . By doing so, I too have gained spiritual strength. I can only thank you for making my friend's last days bearable when once they were unendurable.

The other history follows:

> Mr. John G., aged 61, a self-employed retailer of wine-making supplies, came to St. Christopher's Hospice with a history from his doctor of 18 months of severe spinal pain from a carcinoma of the bronchus unrelieved by laminectomy, radiotherapy, and increasing doses of morphine and chlorpromazine. He knew that he was terminally ill, and both he and his family were feeling exhausted and bitter after months of obviously intense suffering. His drugs

were not altered for the first 48 hr because he began to respond immediately to the atmosphere of security and friendly activity in the ward. After a few days a combination of anti-inflammatory drugs (prednisolone and phenylbutazone) produced a dramatic change in pain and mood. The 4-hourly dose of oral morphine was reduced *from 150 mg to 120 mg,* where it remained. Mr. G. took part fully in the life of the ward; he organized the raffle of a toy made by his sister and began occupational therapy. Two weeks later he was less well and was often drowsy and occasionally somewhat confused, but he continued to enjoy frequent visits from his family and visits to the Hospice bar. He was entirely clear-headed when he sent for his family and announced to them that he did not think he would be alive the next day. He handed over his raffle to another patient, thanked all the staff, and had farewell drinks with his family before he lapsed into unconsciousness and died peacefully 36 hours after he had called them in.

After his death his wife wrote to the ward: "I thank you from the bottom of my heart for the kindness, compassion and caring which you gave to my dear husband. The last month of his life was an unexpected bonus, which turned out to be *pain-free,* care-free and restored his faith—I would add—mine also. I will never forget—God Bless you all."

In both of these case histories, what is noteworthy is that dejected and even dehumanized patients suffering great pain were able to spend the last weeks of their lives in relative comfort and regained much of their previous interest and enjoyment of life. In the case of Mr. G., the dosage of morphine was fifteen times the usual amount prescribed, and even though his illness was progressing and his pain presumably should have become more severe, the dosage could be reduced, and he became pain free as a result of judicious treatment and a greatly improved environment.

In this connection, it has been remarked that improvement in the patient's emotional situation as a result of the comforting community environment contributes significantly to the effectiveness of the drugs used to control pain.

In conclusion, although cancer continues to be one of the major causes of death, much of the fear it inspires would be dispelled if appropriate treatment and care of the types described were more generally available and if the public were better informed on these points.

REFERENCES

Bonica, J.J. Cancer Pain. In Pain *Res. Pub. Assoc. Res. Nerv. Ment. Dis.* 58: 335–362, 1980.

Gerbershagen, H.U. Blocks with local anesthetics in the treatment of cancer pain. *Advances in Pain Research and Therapy* 2: 311–323, 1979.

Saunders, C. The nature and management of terminal pain and the hospice concept. In *Advances in Pain Research and Therapy* 2: 635–651, 1979.

Twycross, R.G. The Brompton cocktail. In *Advances in Pain Research and Therapy* (Ed. by J.J. Bonica and V. Ventafridda). New York: Raven Press, 1979, pp. 291–300.

7

Internal Pain

The internal organs are capable of calling attention to the fact that something has gone wrong by means of pain signals that are often of excruciating intensity. The breath-catching pain of a heart attack and the agonizing, cramping pains that arise from obstruction of the bowel or ureter are typical examples of visceral pain.

Though extremely distressing in many cases, such pains have a value that cannot be overemphasized, for they frequently provide the only warning signal of impending disaster; see, for example, the case of the girl with congenital insensitivity to pain in Chapter 8. For the physician, their characteristics, together with other signs and symptoms, help to establish a diagnosis of the cause of the pain and lead to the implementation of appropriate treatment. In the following pages, some of the more typical patterns of visceral pain are set forth together with appropriate responses that can be instituted.

Pain of Heart Attack: Angina Pectoris

The pain of angina pectoris, or, in more technical terms, the pain that results from a spasm or obstruction of a coronary artery, often has quite a sudden onset. Though the heart is centered mainly in the left side of the chest at and below the nipple, the pain is not felt specifically in that area. Instead, it is felt behind the sternum or breastbone, along the inside of the arm, mainly on the left, often up the left neck, and even into the jaw. It is usually described as a very severe cramping, crushing sensation that may make the victim gasp for breath; nausea, light-headedness, and a feeling of impending death are common, and fainting may occur.

Pain is the result of insufficient blood supply to the heart muscle and is comparable to what develops when a tourniquet is applied tightly to an arm and one continues to exercise it. Very shortly a severe, aching, cramping sensation is felt in the muscles, and soon the pain becomes unbearable. The heart, however, cannot stop to rest, and consequently the pain increases rapidly till it is of great severity. The actual mechanism is that the main trunk or a branch of one of the two coronary arteries that supply the heart muscle becomes obstructed, either by a small clot or by narrowing of its lumen due to fatty deposits in its wall. A variable degree of spasmodic contraction of the affected artery may occur without actual obstruction; this aggravates the problem of already impaired blood supply in the territory of the damaged or partially obstructed artery. From the area of the heart deprived of blood, volleys of pain-producing impulses are discharged centrally along the visceral nerves that form an abundant network around the heart and connect it to the spinal cord. When they reach the centers of consciousness, they are interpreted as arising from the areas I referred to earlier—that is, behind the breastbone, in the arms, and in the neck rather than from the heart itself. This peculiarity, whereby a pain that originates in an internal organ is mistakenly interpreted as arising from an entirely different site, is called "referred pain." Every physician and all patients who have suffered from it are fully aware of its significance; the diagnosis of the affected organ can usually be arrived at in good part from the distribution pattern of the pain. There are, of course, occasions on which the location of the referred pain is quite atypical and thus tends to be misleading.

Control of Cardiac Pain. When the pain is due mainly to spasm of the coronary arteries rather than to total obstruction, drugs that relax the smooth muscle of the vessels are very effective. Amyl nitrite and nitroglycerin have been the drugs of choice for many years; relief is noted within a few seconds to a minute or so after inhaling the former or taking a tablet of the latter under the tongue. However, the effect is as transient as it is rapid, and the need for a longer-lasting coronary antispasmodic drug has long been recognized; this limitation can be offset to a considerable degree by giving larger doses or sustained-release forms of the drugs.

The introduction of Molsidomine, a drug developed in West Germany by the Hoechst Company, appears to be a significant advance in therapy; it is reported to be as effective as nitroglycerin, and its action lasts for up to six hours.

Abdominal Pain—Stomachaches

To use a rather hackneyed expression, the causes of abdominal pain are legion; an attempt to condense so vast a subject would be futile and would almost certainly give the reader an inadequate and unbalanced view. As a general rule, any acute pain that lasts for more than an hour or two, any sudden severe pain, or any pain of mild to moderate intensity that tends to persist or become chronic, should be investigated by a physician. In most instance common sense will be the best guide; when in doubt, see a physician, since a significant number of abdominal pains prove to be early warning signals of disease. Others, on the other hand, are of little or no significance. I limit my comments to two fairly common types of abdominal pain that may cause considerable, but usually unfounded, anxiety.

Stomachache in Children. Between the ages of five and fifteen this is a common complaint, and about 10 percent of youngsters with this problem will have recurrent episodes of pain over periods of months or years.

Apley (1975) has surveyed this problem in considerable detail in an excellent monograph entitled *The Child with Abdominal Pain,* on which the following description is based in good part. The pain that is described as a dull ache, colicky, or sharp and pinching is severe in about a quarter, moderate in a quarter, and mild in half of the cases and is located around the umbilicus. It lasts for a few moments, is succeeded by a pain-free period of several minutes, and is followed by another bout of pain. The whole episode may be over quite rapidly, but sometimes it may last for several hours and rarely for a day or two. Pallor, nausea, vomiting, headache, and/or loss of appetite are common accompaniments. Because of its characteristics and its localization around the umbilicus, it is thought that the pain may be due to spasm of the small intestine or possibly of the stomach.

What Is the Cause? Apley, who is one of the authorities on this problem, notes that when he first became interested in it, his inclination was to believe that it had an organic basis—that is, that infection of some type or perhaps a toxic factor might be responsible. Careful investigation of many children with stomachache has convinced him—and others—that the vast majority of cases are due to emotional problems such as anxiety about an impending examination, parental quarrels, and so on. Thus, of 100 children with recurrent episodes of stomachache, only eight had an identifiable organic basis for their complaint; four of these had a disorder of the urinary system and not of the abdominal viscera at all!

What to Do? Although the most logical approach would seem to be to give the child an antispasmodic drug to suppress the intestinal cramping, experience has indicated that the best results are obtained by reassurance and conditioning techniques that help the child to overcome his or her anxieties and misgivings rather than trying to abolish the end result of this process.

Once again, when in doubt about abdominal pain, and especially if it is severe or prolonged, one should seek medical advice; even then, in some instances it may be very difficult to establish a diagnosis of the cause.

"Stomach" Ulcer Pain. "My ulcer is acting up" has become a commonplace expression that appears to be indiscriminately applied to almost any abdominal discomfort. In actual fact, there are many causes of abdominal discomfort and pain unrelated to ulcers. Thus, acute gastritis due to unaccustomed or contaminated foods, simple hypersecretion of gastric acid, or reflux of acid with a burning sensation up behind the sternum, or heartburn, are quite common minor disorders. The syndrome of stomach ulcers is (1) not due to an ulcer of the stomach in most cases and (2) usually has rather characteristic features that help to establish the diagnosis.

Actually, duodenal ulcers are at the root of most of the ulcer syndromes. The pain is usually felt in the mid and upper part of the abdomen, and it is usually of a cramping or pressure type. It often extends horizontally like a band and, very typically, is aggravated by fasting. For this reason, it usually appears an hour or two after meals and, characteristically, is promptly alleviated by drinking a glass of milk or taking an antacid tablet. Another feature is that ulcer pain occurs in a periodic manner, being present daily for several weeks to disappear for a few months and then recur, a pattern that may repeat for years.

A sudden severe increase in the pain may indicate that a perforation has occurred, and similarly, a change in the distribution of the pain may also be a warning that it has progressed and invaded an adjacent organ such as the pancreas. Acute or persistent abdominal pain should be taken seriously and medical advice obtained without delay, since a life-threatening situation may be developing.

Pelvic Pain

Inflammatory and tumoral disorders of the uterus and related organs (ovaries, Fallopian tubes) are the source of much of the pain experienced in the pelvis by women. The details of diagnosis and treatment of these conditions are beyond the scope of this chapter, but some comments regarding dysmenorrhea, a common benign painful syndrome, are of interest.

The pain is usually of a cramping or colicky type but may be a continuous dull ache. Located mainly in the lower abdomen, it often radiates to the hip joints, the low back, and the legs. Though it may begin at any time after puberty, it is most common after the age of eighteen, and is characteristically related to the menstrual period.

About 40 to 50 percent of women in the childbearing period are affected by it, and its more severe forms can be incapacitating. In some instances it is caused by a benign lesion called endometriosis or by scarring of the uterine adnexa, but commonly there is no pathology.

The factor responsible for this uncomplicated variety, or "primary dysmenorrhea," is now known to be an overproduction of prostaglandins by the uterus, as first established by Pickering and associates of Sheffield University, England. Subsequent studies have fully confirmed their conclusions, and the introduction of a series of potent inhibitors of prostaglandin synthesis such as indomethacin, mefenamic acid, fenoprofen calcium, ibuprofen, and naproxen sodium now provides the first effective means of relieving and even completely suppressing this painful and very distressing disorder. At this time, however, although these drugs are approved for the treatment of arthritis, they are not approved by the FDA for the control of dysmenorrheic pain.

CHILDBIRTH

For centuries, pain was regarded as an inevitable accompaniment of childbirth; only with the advent of general anesthesia could women, for the first time, be assured that if major discomfort developed during delivery, they need not suffer. Even so, there were those who claimed that childbirth pains were "God's will" or "nature's way," that therefore they were good for the woman, and that anesthesia was quite unnecessary.

These endlessly repeated, ignorant opinions, together with a potpourri of superstitions, made childbirth something many women dreaded; perhaps quite a few men would be, shall we say appalled, were they to have to deliver something the size of a full term baby through their perinea.* True, the male pelvis is narrower than that of the female, but it is still a remarkable fact of nature that the process can take place at all.

The degree of pain and discomfort that occurs during labor—the preliminary phase during which uterine contractions, progressive descent of the baby, and dilatation of the cervix take place—and delivery varies considerably, and it depends on many factors. For example, in some unsophisticated societies, childbirth is taken so casually that it is common for a pregnant woman working in the fields to leave her chores for a couple of hours or less and return to them with her newborn. This is by no means to be taken as evidence that she does not experience pain, but rather that her attitude toward delivery and pain is different.

Conversely, in the more affluent societies, attitudes toward childbirth are more complex. For some women, it is a rewarding, exciting, and deeply

---

**Perineum:* The area between the thighs that contains the anus and the genitalia.

fulfilling experience that they look forward to and enjoy. For others, just the opposite is the case; they approach the event with fear and revulsion and consider it to be one of the burdens of womanhood that have to be endured. Far from being an enjoyable experience, for them, it is painful, exhausting, and thoroughly unpleasant, and some vow never to go through with it again after a single discouraging delivery. Obviously, between these two extremes, there are a great number of women whose emotional reactions are intermediate.

As in other types of situations in which pain may be a significant factor, it is helpful to understand something about the mechanisms involved in order to deal with the experience in a well-balanced and assured manner. The unfounded lore and consequent fears about childbirth never wilt faster than when they are exposed to simple logical facts.

Mechanism of Labor Pains

Once the fetus has reached full term, a variety of glandular and nervous mechanisms come into play that result in intermittent contractions of the uterus of gradually increasing frequency and intensity. These contractions have two major outcomes. One of these is that the baby is squeezed downward, deeper into the pelvis. This is because it is the only direction in which it can go and because the muscular uterine sack is attached to the lower and lateral parts of the pelvis. The other effect is that the cervix—which is normally somewhat like a champagne cork in shape and size, with a small canal running through its center—is gradually stretched and thinned out, as its muscle is pulled on by the rest of the uterus; later, the uterine contents, under pressure, wedge into and against it. This is the process of dilatation, which is, of course, necessary if the head and body of the baby are to emerge.

As this sequence of events develops, the pressure on the pelvis increases progressively, and the ligaments between the pelvic bones at the front and between these bones and the sacrum at the back, are progressively stretched. Because of endocrine changes that have occurred in the last few months of pregnancy, these ligaments have become considerably softer and more lax than usual, so that the separation occurs without excessive strain; that it is a valuable phenomenon is undoubted, since every additional fraction of an inch in diameter of the pelvic canal makes childbirth that much easier and less traumatic for both mother and child.

With regard to the pain that occurs throughout this period, some obstetricians believe that it is not due to the contractions themselves but that it occurs immediately after them, whereas others hold the opposite opinion. Whatever its precise origin, there is no doubt that pain does occur, usually in the mid and lower abdomen; frequently there is a deep, dull, aching pain felt particularly in the small of the back, in the kidney area. Some of the pain appears to come from the uterine muscle itself and some from the surrounding attachments and organs, which are supplied with an extremely rich network of sensory fibers. It is, therefore, not surprising that pain should be felt during this complex combination of stretching, pulling, and compression.

Is Pain Useful in Labor?

With this question, we can go back to my earlier comment about the unenlightened opinions of those who, in an earlier age, claimed that the pain served a useful purpose. Today we have evidence that far from being useful, labor pains may actually be harmful, especially to the baby.

According to Bonica (1972), the rapid breathing induced by the pain the pregnant mother feels results in loss of acidity of her blood (alkalosis), and this in turn leads to constriction of the uterine arterioles. Pain also induces the release of agents (catecholamines) that produce further constriction of blood vessels. This combination of factors impairs the blood supply of the uterus and may consequently have an unfavorable influence on the fetus, which receives its blood supply from the uterus via the placenta. Bonica, furthermore, points out that in those instances in which a complication occurs during delivery, the impairment in fetal blood supply may be a decisive factor in determining the death of the fetus.

Childbirth Without Pain

Nowadays, labor pains should no longer be a source of anxiety and foreboding to prospective mothers, since a variety of effective and safe methods of pain control are readily available. These range from general and spinal anesthesia to hypnosis and "natural" childbirth. Each of these methods has advantages and disadvantages, either for the mother or the baby or both; which one is selected will depend on the obstetrician and/or anesthesiologist, and, in some instances, maternal preference.

Anesthesia. Anesthetic methods include general anesthesia, discussed in Chapter 9, and the now much more popular method of lumbar epidural anesthetic blockade. This consists of injecting an anesthetic solution into the spinal canal around the dura mater without entering the spinal fluid (see page 62, Chapter 5, for descriptions of these compartments). This method suppresses pain and has little or no adverse effect on the newborn.

A new method of suppressing pain has been introduced recently by Yaksh and associates (1979). A very small amount of morphine—about one-tenth the usual dose—is injected into the spinal fluid by lumbar puncture. This suppresses pain sensations while sparing motor and reflex functions; the effect lasts for some eight to sixteen hours. It is still too early to know whether this will prove to be superior to methods currently in use, but the very small amount of morphine required as well as the preservation of motor functions and thus of the expulsive action of the uterus are very attractive features.

To this point, chemical methods of suppressing pain have been described; these have been used for over a hundred years with ever-increasing effectiveness and safety, so that today complications due to anesthesia are infrequent. However, it can be, and frequently is, argued that the use of drugs should be avoided in view of their potentially deleterious effects on the fetus. This point of view is especially persuasive when its sponsors can show that alternative methods that do not require administration of drugs can provide pain-free childbirth. How successful are these alternatives, and what are their limitations, if any?

Hypnosis. Hypnosis has been used sporadically for the control of pain in childbirth since the early days of the nineteenth century. For a variety of reasons, and especially because of the relative difficulty of obtaining an adequate hypnotic state in a considerable proportion of the population (see Chapter 13), it has failed to gain widespread acceptance.

"Natural" Childbirth

In the last thirty years or so, "natural" childbirth has become quite popular in the Western world, particularly among the more sophisticated segments of the population. Since the method is frequently employed and is claimed by its supporters to result in childbirth without pain, it is of some interest to review briefly what it is and what results can be expected of it.

The method was first described by the English obstetrician Dick-Read in 1933 and was based on his hypothesis that women experience pain during childbirth because they have been conditioned by society to expect it. He believed that apprehension resulted in exaggerated contractions of the uterus during labor and that this in turn led to pain. This emotional state was, in his opinion, further aggravated by the loneliness of the woman in labor, the impersonal attitude of attendants, and the strangeness of the hospital environment. Dick-Read's method of combating these negative influences was to explain to potential mothers that childbirth need not be painful and to dissipate the unwarranted fears arising from superstition and folklore.

Similar to this are the methods of psychoprophylaxis developed by Velvovsky (1960) in Russia and Lamaze (1970) in France; however, in addition to providing expectant mothers with correct information on childbirth, a series of breathing exercises are taught, whose objective is to help the woman to relax and improve the oxygenation of her blood.

Evaluation of "Natural" Childbirth. The first issue that should be raised is what precisely is meant by "natural" childbirth. Presumably this type of childbirth should be found in its purest form among underdeveloped societies. However, those who have actually practiced midwifery among primitive peoples and who have evaluated the reports of others who have investigated the subject (see M. Stanton 1979) have concluded quite unequivocally that there is no such thing as natural childbirth among these peoples. Not only do they surround delivery with a variety of rites, physical maneuvers, and administration of drugs, but pain is usually associated with the process. Going further, there is some evidence that even in monkeys, parturition is associated with a degree of suffering (Tinklepaugh and Hartman, 1930); certainly there is no reason to believe that female monkeys are somehow led to expect that they will have labor pains! The socially induced expectation of pain theory seems, thus, to have little basis in fact. In summary, "natural" childbirth in the context in which it is commonly used appears to be a misnomer and to have little relationship to reality.

On the other hand, a large number of favorable reports in the obstetric literature and in the lay press suggest that "natural" childbirth not only decreases or suppresses pain and thus the amount of analgesic drugs required, but that it also decreases blood loss, operative procedures, and the duration of labor. However, when Beck and Hall of the Missouri Medical School made an exhaustive analysis (1978) of all the published reports on psychoprophylaxis up to October 1977, they concluded that it was impossible to reach any definitive conclusions about its value in view of the inadequate design of the studies. Their summarizing comment will perhaps give the reader a better feel for the situation than a more detailed discussion of each issue. As they put it:

> On the whole, it is difficult to recall an obstetric issue that has remained so controversial for such an extended period of time . . . it has been acclaimed as one of the most significant advances of modern medicine and as a primitive and medically unacceptable practice. Even more disturbing than the polarization [of opinion] itself is the fact that this process has occurred in the absence of a single adequately controlled study of therapeutic outcome.

There are, of course, a considerable number of women who have borne children without any significant discomfort using these methods. This raises the question of placebo effect and emotional overtones. As noted repeatedly throughout this book, the affective state of an individual at any given time determines to a great extent just how tolerable pain will be.

Many factors influence the emotional state; the reassurance and soothing effects of psychoprophylaxis together with the more or less convincing manner of the person conducting the lectures and the receptiveness and confidence of the expectant mother may be the major factors leading to the creation of a joyful experience for those who find "natural" childbirth successful.

ARTHRITIS AND PAIN

Pain from disorders that affect the joints and surrounding tissues is one of the commonest of complaints. It is estimated that in the United States alone, some 20 million people suffer from some form of arthritis; the cumulative misery and disruption of life-style is incalculable; loss of income and cost of treatment is estimated at $10 billion per annum, according to the National Institute of Arthritis, Metabolism and Digestive Diseases.

As a generalization, arthritis can be of two main varieties: One of these results from inflammation of the joint tissues, which become swollen, hot, and painful; the most common types are rheumatoid arthritis and gout. The other variety of arthritis is due to degeneration of the joint surfaces associated with bony overgrowth but without any overt signs of inflammation; this is called *osteoarthritis* and tends to affect older people. These and the other less frequent types of arthritis have in common a tendency to chronicity, and their major symptom is pain.

Rheumatoid Arthritis

Rheumatoid arthritis is a disease of unknown cause that may begin at any age and can affect any joint and any number of joints simultaneously. The soft (synovial) membrane that encloses the joint cavity becomes swollen and infiltrated with inflammatory cells, and the nerve fibers within it become sensitized so that even slight movement produces pain. The inflammation of the synovial membrane results in an increase in secretion of fluid into the joint, which further distends the joint cavity and increases pain. Soft tissues surrounding the joint are also involved, and the sum total of swelling gives the joint a puffy appearance. The joints of the fingers are often the first to be affected, and thereafter other joints become involved at intervals. Interestingly, there are often symptom-free periods of months or even years, and in some cases a single episode may occur without any subsequent recurrence. In most cases, however, the disease advances relentlessly, and progressive degenerative changes of the joint surface together with scarring of the soft tissues around the joint result in gradual loss of mobility and crippling.

Gout

Gout is a metabolic disorder in which uric acid, a product of the breakdown of proteins, precipitates as crystals in joints. An inflammatory response results, with swelling of the soft tissues, heat, and pain. As in other types of arthritis, the basic cause of gout is unknown. Certain joints are more susceptible to gouty involvement than others; the most typically affected is the joint at the base of the big toe.

Osteoarthritis

Osteoarthritis, the noninflammatory degenerative joint disease, also of unknown cause, is characterized by progressive breakdown of the smooth cartilage of the joints, which becomes roughened and pitted. Fragments of the cartilage may break off and lie loose in the joint cavity. Simultaneously, abnormal so-called reactive bony growth occurs around the joint, with the production of excrescences and spurlike formations. The most severely affected joints are the hips and knees because of the amount of weight they bear. Typically, it is an arthritis of aging, but this alone is not a sufficient explanation for the degenerative changes, since many aged individuals have few or no symptoms of joint pain. Injury to the joints from excessive physical exertion or related to certain occupations is an important contributor in some instances, but why joint breakdown is so much more severe in some people than in others is still an enigma.

Treatment of the Pain

Because of the likelihood of serious disability resulting from inadequately treated arthritis, it is absolutely imperative that any joint pain that lasts for more than a week to ten days or any severe joint pain, regardless of the brevity of its duration, receive careful medical examination and treatment. Although it is true that one can self-medicate mild joint pains, this is at the risk of inadequate dosage and/or of allowing the disorder to progress, under cover of pain suppression, to the point where serious or even irreversible damage has occurred.

One of the most effective means of dealing with arthritis is rest, particularly during acute flare-ups. These may require complete bed rest when several joints are involved or simply taking the pressure off affected weight-bearing joints.

Aspirin and related compounds, such as sodium salicylate, are effective drugs for treating arthritis. In the case of the inflammatory types of arthritis, aspirin is particularly effective because it not only alleviates pain but also has a significant anti-inflammatory action that reduces the swelling and infiltration of soft tissues. The effective dosages of aspirin are usually high, and because of the danger of toxic side effects, treatment should be under the supervision of a physician. Several new and powerful nonnarcotic analgesics are now available for treating this type of pain (see Chapter 10).

The use of adrenocortical steroids such as cortisone and related preparations can be of great value in suppressing a flare-up and preventing acute damage to joints. However, these powerful drugs have a number of undesirable side effects and must be administered under close supervision by a physician.

Physiotherapy is invaluable in maintaining joint mobility and muscle strength while helping to rehabilitate the patient with limited use of a joint.

One of the greatest boons to patients with pain and severe impairment of joint function is the development of artificial joints. First introduced as the "total hip arthroplasty," almost any diseased joint can now be replaced with a high degree of success. As one author noted, this is probably the greatest advance in prosthetic replacement to date. The complete disappearance of pain and restoration of virtually normal function cannot be achieved by any other means. Complications such as loosening of the prosthesis and infection of the operated area occur infrequently.

REFERENCES

Abdominal Pain

APLEY, J. *The child with abdominal pain* (2nd ed.). Oxford: Blackwell Scientific, 1975.

Childbirth

BECK, N.C., and HALL, D. Natural childbirth: A review and analysis. *Obstetrics and Gynecology* 52: 371–379, 1978.

BONICA, J.J. Maternal respiratory changes during pregnancy and parturition. In *Parturition and Perinatology* (Ed. by G. F. Marx). Philadelphia: F. A. Davis, 1972, pp. 1–19.

DICK-READ, G. *Natural childbirth.* London: W. Heinemann, 1933.

LAMAZE, F. *Painless childbirth. Psychoprophylactic method* (Transl. by L. R. Clestin). Chicago: Regnery, 1970, 192 pp.

STANTON, M.E. The myth of "natural" childbirth. *Journal of Nurse-Midwifery* 24: 25–29, 1979.

TINKLEPAUGH, O.L. and HARTMAN, C.G. Behavioral aspects of parturition in the monkey (macacus rhesus). *Journal of Comparative Psychology* 11: 63–97, 1930.

VELVOVSKY, I.Z., et al. *Painless childbirth through psychoprophylaxis* (Transl. D. A. Myshne). Moscow: Foreign Language Pub. House, 1960.

YAKSH, T.L.; WILSON, P.R.; KAIKO, R.F.; and INTURRISI, C.E. Analgesia produced by a spinal action of morphine and effects upon parturition in the rat. *Anesthesiology* 51: 386–392, 1979.

Arthritis

Out of the Maze. Vol. 1. *The Arthritis Plan.* National Commission on Arthritis and Related Muskuloskeletal Diseases. Report to the Congress of the United States, Department of Health, Education and Welfare, April 1976.

HOLLANDER, J. L. (Ed.). *The arthritis handbook: A problem-solving approach to arthritis management.* West Point, Pa.: Merck, Sharp & Dohme, 1974, 178 pp.

WOLFF, B.B. Arthritis and rheumatism. In *Rehabilitation practices with the physically disabled* (Ed. by J. F. Garrett and E. S. Levine.) New York: Columbia University Press, 1973, pp. 336–397.

8

No Pain and Spontaneous Pain

Whether a stimulus will be felt as pain or not depends, on one hand, on its nature and intensity and, on the other, on the condition of the nervous system of the subject. Provided the latter is functioning normally, nonnoxious stimuli will be perceived as touch—warm, cold, rough, and so on; whereas noxious stimuli will be perceived as pain—sharp, hot, cramping, and the like.

This comment is so obvious as to seem trite, but if we analyze it a bit more closely, it soon becomes evident that normal function implies a vast number of qualifying factors. The system is set to respond as soon as threshold (see Chapter 1) is reached and then to sort out, screen out, accept, or reject and then relay, analyze, and finally decide whether the stimulus is desirable, undesirable, or to be ignored. Once this stage is reached, and it only takes a fraction of a second for all this processing to be done, a response is made. Sometimes, however, the system has suffered damage and misinterprets the signals. The result may then be chaotic and even life threatening.

The two main possibilities that can occur are that noxious stimuli are not perceived as such or, conversely, that nonnoxious stimuli are interpreted as being painful—indeed, excruciatingly painful; that is, either too little or too much response occurs. Too little is just as undesirable as too much, and we first look at the result of this in a condition called congenital insensitivity to pain.

TOO LITTLE: CONGENITAL INSENSITIVITY TO PAIN

Congenital insensitivity to pain is a very rare disorder, only a small number of cases having been reported in the world literature; a typical example follows:

Annie was three years old when her mother first noticed that she would bump herself quite violently without ever complaining or, indeed, showing the least sign of discomfort. She was particularly taken aback one winter day when her daughter leaned against the hot metal of a wood-burning stove and burned herself severely but neither cried out nor complained. Because of serious blistering, she was taken to a doctor, who dressed the injury and pointed out that the child had numerous scars as well as bite marks on her tongue and lips and lacerations in her nose. Though she was eight years old at the time of her visit to the doctor, she acted as if she were a much younger child, and it was evident that she had a mild degree of mental deficiency.

She continued to damage herself on repeated occasions, and at age twelve, she fractured her ankle and, as usual, felt no pain. One afternoon during her sixteenth year, she became nauseated and languid and vomited several times. She was put to bed, but the following day she had a high fever, and her condition was so grave that a physician was called urgently. Immediate operation was advised, and a gangrenous, perforated appendix was removed. The striking feature of this episode was that at no time did she have any abdominal discomfort whatsoever from what is normally a very painful condition and, as a result, very nearly lost her life.

This story is fairly typical of one type of congenital insensitivity to pain in that it is present from birth; multiple painless injuries occur, some of which may be self-inflicted, as in the case of the bite injuries to her lips and tongue and the lacerations in her nose due to her frequent picking at it until it bled. Mental deficiency may or may not be present, and one or more of the child's brothers or sisters may also be affected. Although some of these people have degenerative changes in their peripheral nerves or in the central nervous system, in others no changes are found; and it has been proposed that they have a mental inability to conceptualize pain, or what has been termed *asymbolia* for pain. The latter, however, is exceedingly rare, and when it does occur, it is believed to be due to damage to the parietal cortex of the brain.

What congenital insensitivity to pain illustrates so well is the importance of pain as a normal protective system that is constantly on watch; not only does it help to avoid injuries, but on occasion it may give a life-saving warning. The value of pain in many other situations is clearly apparent; it prevents us from moving a fractured limb, thus avoiding further damage to the bone and soft tissues; it stops the victim of angina pectoris from moving, thus reducing stress on the heart and possibly saving a life; and it alerts us to impending danger from inflammation, tumors, and other diseases and gets us to the hospital in time.

Congenital insensitivity to pain is not the only condition in which pain is absent, however; profound loss of sensation may occur in leprosy, a disease that is almost nonexistent in the more technologically advanced countries and that is slowly disappearing from the rest of the world. In one form of leprosy, the organism invades nerves, and as a result, progressive loss of sensation occurs in the areas supplied by the affected nerve. Loss of sensation results in repeated injuries to fingers and other parts of the body; infection and ulceration set in, and loss of tissue occurs. It is probable that some of the remarkable demonstrations of insensibility to pain by fakirs and holy men are better attributed to leprosy than to divine inspiration!

Even more selective than leprosy in abolishing pain is syringomyelia, an infrequent disease that cores out a cavity in or near the center of the spinal cord. As it does so, it destroys fibers of the "pain pathway," leaving other sensations such as touch and pressure intact. Patients with this disease also burn and otherwise damage themselves and may, as a result, suffer serious injuries.

TOO MUCH: WHEN THE SEAT OF PAIN IS MAINLY IN THE BRAIN, OR CENTRAL PAIN

In the preceding examples, sensitivity to injury was impaired, the system was negatively affected, and patients were, so to speak, protected from the unpleasantness that this sensation evokes. But at what cost!—ulcerations, burns, fractures, and even the risk of death.

As we speculate about the causes of pain, our thoughts naturally center on burns, mechanical injuries, inflammations (toothache, peritonitis, pleurisy), or cancer. All of these are obvious and well-known sources of pain, and the cause-and-effect relationship seems quite logical, even though we may not fully understand how some of these pains are actually engendered.

Rarely, if ever, does a nonspecialist consider that pain in a limb, the face—indeed, anywhere in the body—may be due, not to any local factor, but instead to some disorder in the nervous system itself. Nevertheless, there are a number of situations in which damage to the brain, either by mechanical injury, a surgical procedure, a stroke, or a tumor, may result in pain of the most incapacitating and intractable nature.

An example of this most distressing of pains is that of a fifty-four-year-old woman who had had hypertension for several years. Shortly after breakfast one day, she noted some clumsiness of her left arm and leg; this progressed to the point where she had to lie down, and she then found that "the strength had gone from all her left side." She was slightly confused and complained of a moderately severe headache in the back of her head. At a nearby hospital she was told that she had had a stroke: a hemorrhage into the right side of her brain due to high blood pressure that had ruptured a small artery. Over the ensuing weeks her left-sided paralysis improved considerably, and she was able to get up and around, at first with the aid of a walker and later with a cane. She noted some blunting of sensation on her left side, but toward the end of the third week after her stroke, she began to have pains of a very peculiar and unpleasant nature in her arm. These consisted in quite severe burning sensations in the skin; touching and especially light stroking of her arm markedly aggravated these sensations, much as stroking aggravates the pain of a recent severe sunburn. Not only was this very distressing, since it required her to avoid contact with her arm, but it was also very puzzling to her, since sensation on her left side had been severely impaired from the beginning. After a couple of weeks the burning pain was present almost constantly and was aggravated, as before, by mechanical contact, so that she could not bear to have the bed sheets touch her. Sometimes, without any stimulus, she would experience sudden, quite violent burning and stabbing pains on her left side that made her cry out. None of the analgesic drugs gave her any relief from the pain, which continued in much the same way for two months; at that time she had another stroke that was much more severe and from which she did not recover.

This story is fairly characteristic of thalamic pain, one of several types of central pain; fortunately, it is a relatively infrequent complication of a stroke, since on one hand, acute vascular damage to the brain due to occlusion or rupture of blood vessels is very common, and on the other, there is very little that can be done to alleviate central pain. As if it were not enough that the pain is often unbearable and responds poorly or not at all to drug therapy, it tends to continue indefinitely, transforming the patient's life into an unending martyrdom. Such patients, as can well be imagined, become severely depressed, querulous, and withdrawn; some of them commit suicide as the only way out of their predicament.

What Is the Reason for Such Pains?

No generally accepted explanation for spontaneous pain of this type has been formulated yet, and as a result, theories and speculation abound. The most likely cause is that the hemorrhage or other lesions destroy a part of the thalamus (see Chapter 2) that is concerned with modulating noxious input while the neurons that signal pain are preserved. The latter, being released from control, fire in a disorderly, hyperexcitable manner, and the patient perceives this as pain. The reason for believing this is that in carefully conducted studies of the brains of patients with thalamic pain who have succumbed, most of the thalamus (see Chapter 2), including much of the pain relay areas, has been spared; whereas the damaged area tends to involve the posterior part of this nucleus, which is related mainly to mechanical rather than noxious signaling.

One might look upon central pain, then, as a kind of runway discharge of pain relay neurons that are no longer under the control of the normal braking or balancing system. Expressed in other terms, in the normal functioning of the nervous system, there is always a delicately adjusted balance between excitation and inhibition. When inhibition or the braking system is damaged, excitation predominates; if it is in the motor system, convulsions or epilepsy result, whereas in the sensory system, exaggerated and abnormal sensations occur (so-called hyperesthesiae and painful paresthesiae, respectively). As I mentioned previously, other hypotheses have been offered to account for the disordered pain mechanisms; rather than list them, I provide references at the end of the chapter with greater detail for the reader desirous of further information.

Is There Anything That Can Be Done?

Since drug treatment of central pain has been unsuccessful, what if anything can be offered to the unfortunate victims of this harrowing disorder? When drugs fail, resort to surgery has been common; it must be remembered, in this respect, that patients in this situation are desperate for relief and that in the face of so much suffering, it is difficult, if not frankly inhuman, for the physician or surgeon to maintain a detached attitude. Thus, procedures that would normally be regarded as too hazardous to merit consideration may have to be entertained.

Over the years a number of operations were tried, ranging from psychosurgery to stereotaxic thalamotomies (see Chapter 11). The results were disappointing since only an occasional patient benefited. Some encouragement may be derived now from the development of stimulus-produced analgesia (SPA), or so-called neuroaugmentative operations, discussed in Chapter 11. Insofar as central pain is concerned, some successes have been reported; the operation consists in introducing an electrode into a discrete area of the brain by means of a stereotaxic guidance system and then stimulating a selected area around its tip. The risks of the procedure are small compared to the gravity of the problem, and a number of patients have had enduring relief; this, of course, requires long-term intermittent stimulation, but there is little doubt that it constitutes an encouraging advance in an otherwise intractable and gloomy area of human pain.

OTHER TYPES OF CENTRAL PAIN

Damage to any one of a number of sites in the central nervous system can result in chronic, intractable pain. Again, such pain syndromes are relatively uncommon, but like the one resulting from damage to the thalamus, they are extremely difficult to treat. Here, I limit my comments to brief descriptions of some of these syndromes, since detailed discussion is more appropriate for specialized treatises.

Injuries of the spinal cord as a result of a fractured back, for example, are not infrequently followed by more or less severe pains of a burning or crushing type. The spinal cord may be completely severed, yet the pain is referred to—that is, felt—in the completely anesthetic area of the body below the injured part of the cord. Recutting of the damaged tip of the cord above the transection has not succeeded in relieving the pain for most of these patients, and it is speculated, therefore, that some abnormal pain circuitry has developed at a higher level in the brain.

Occasionally, disagreeable crawling, burning, and frankly painful sensations (dysesthesiae) may develop after a spinal cordotomy (see Chapter 11) has been done to relieve pain.

Injuries of various types to the brain stem—that is, the portion of the central nervous system between the upper end of the spinal cord and the cerebral hemispheres—may also result in chronic intractable pain. One classical example of this was the unexpected outcome of attempts in the 1940s to relieve chronic pain by severing the pain pathway high in the stem—that is, in the mesencephalon. Only a small number of operations of this type were carried out, because the incidence of spontaneous central pain was high—between 60 and 80 percent of cases—making the cure worse than the condition for which it had been devised. The combination of disagreeable crawling, tickling sensations with sharp and/or burning pain was so distressing and so refractory to any type of treatment that several patients committed suicide rather than try to live with it. It is well to emphasize, once again, that such operations were only done as a last resort, in the hope of providing the sufferer with at least a modicum of relief; the disillusion and anguish of the compassionate surgeon in these instances are rarely if ever commented on and can be understood only by those who have had to tread this difficult and unrewarding path.

Several types of injuries of the peripheral nervous system can also produce chronic, severe, spontaneous pain. Of these, phantom limb pain and causalgia are particularly distressing.

Phantom Limb Pain

Amputation of a limb is usually followed by peculiarly vivid sensations that the extremity is still present; sometimes it feels as if the imaginary limb is much larger than normal, bent into an unusual position, or otherwise distorted. The term *phantom limb* has been aptly coined to describe these bizarre illusions. In a few of these patients, the phantom limb may feel as if it is being crushed in a vise, twisted painfully, or otherwise injured. The syndrome is then called *phantom limb pain.*

Treatment for this condition has been very unsatisfactory; one of the few approaches that have been successful on occasion is the placement of minute lesions in the spinal cord where the nociceptive fibers terminate (Nashold, Urban, and Zorub 1976). In some instances, relief has been obtained by stimulus-produced analgesia (SPA), as described in Chapter 11.

Causalgia

> A. F. Swann, aged thirty-four, a native of Pennsylvania, a stout, robust man, and then captain of C Company, 16th Pennsylvania Cavalry, was wounded by a minie-ball at the battle of Cold Harbor, Virginia, May 28, 1864. The ball, fired at about ten rods* distance, entered the forearm two inches below the head of the radius, and passing obliquely across the elbow joint, made its exit just above the inner condyle of the humerus. From the moment he was struck he suffered the most intense pain in the arm and hand, and lost a large quantity of blood.

Thus did Silas Weir Mitchell (1829–1914) introduce one of the soldiers of the War Between the States who suffered from what he called *causalgia,*

*A rod is 5½ yards.

or burning pain, from the Greek (*kausos:* heat; and *algia:* pain). The pain continued unabated, and a month after the injury it was described as excruciating, located mainly in the palm of the hand, and feeling as if a red-hot iron were being grasped. At Captain Swann's insistence, an operation was done to try to relieve his pain, and a three-inch segment of the affected nerve was said to have been removed by a surgeon named Bliss, at Armory Square Hospital, but without success. From that time he took injections of morphine in quantities of up to 10 grains (650 mg) per day.

Weir Mitchell advised another operation in June of 1865, but Captain Swann declined on the advice of a number of physicians who assured him that it too would fail. Five years later he was seen by Weir Mitchell again, at which time

> [h]is condition was most deplorable, the pain in the hand, which was intensified by any excitement was indescribable, and he was unable to attend any active duties, except while under the influence of morphine. He suffered from nervous chills of two or three hours duration, when he would be obliged, in the heat of midsummer, to lie by a hot stove with four or five blankets over him, the cold perspiration, meanwhile streaming from him. His appetite was nearly gone; his bowels were habitually constipated; and the whole man was emaciated and fretful. He was willing to undergo any operation which promised relief, even amputation of the arm.

This story is quoted verbatim from Weir Mitchell's report (1872); it may seem almost unbelievable that a nerve injury could reduce a stout, robust soldier to this pitiful condition; such, however, is the power of unrelenting, intense pain.

Mitchell goes on to describe the operation he then performed on June 27, 1870: Under ether anesthesia, he removed three inches of the median nerve. From the moment the patient awoke, he was entirely free of pain, and this never returned. Most strikingly, he never used opiates again, despite the widespread belief that addiction is invariable after repeated exposure; in this respect Captain Swann's arms were covered with punctures from hypodermic injections—which he received from six to twenty times daily—and were discolored and indurated as a result. In the chapter on drugs (Chapter 10) I have noted this peculiar feature of opiates: Addiction is usual when a person takes the drug for its psychic effects but much less common when pain is the only, or at least the main, reason for medication. The only residual effect of his heavy morphine intake was that he had great difficulty sleeping, insisting that "he scarcely slept an hour for fourteen days [after the operation] and had not a sound night's sleep for twenty-six days after it."

Causalgia, then, is a special type of traumatic nerve lesion, commonly seen in wartime when high-velocity projectiles cause many injuries. The pain may begin immediately, as in the case history described, or its onset may be delayed for hours or days. Characteristically it is a burning, agonizing sensation, often accompanied by sensations of "pins and needles." Though not specifically noted in the case history described, marked changes occur in the appearance of the skin, which becomes glossy and puffy, acquires a mottled, bluish color, and is usually colder than normal, though occasionally it is warmer. So intense is the pain that the victim protects the affected part from the lightest contact; even noises, loud music, or anything startling will aggravate it and precipitate a paroxysm of unbearable agony. Nearly all patients rapidly learn that the one thing that decreases the pain to a slight degree is keeping the part constantly moistened or soaked in cold water. In some patients the pain may decrease spontaneously and disappear after several months, but in others it lasts for years; some of Weir Mitchell's patients from the Civil War still suffered from it in the 1890s, as described by his son.

Mechanism. The most generally accepted view is that the nerve injury permits impulses that go out in sympathetic nerve fibers to find their way into sensory nerve fibers that normally signal noxious events. In other words, a short circuit is established, and spontaneous pain is the result.

Treatment. Weir Mitchell reported that cures could be obtained in some instances by blistering the skin, whereas in intractable cases he resected an extensive portion of the damaged nerve and met with considerable success. This, of course, resulted in both anesthesia and paralysis of the area supplied by the affected nerve; however, when the patient's desperation had reached the point where he begged for anything that might give relief, including amputation, it was not unreasonable to excise a long segment of the nerve. Such a radical procedure is, fortunately, no longer necessary, since it was shown during World War II that interrupting the sympathetic supply to the involved extremity gives a very high percentage of lasting cures.

To conclude this chapter, the examples of loss of pain sensation show how valuable this sensory function is; overreaction to pain, on the other hand—whether due to central or peripheral nerve disorders—may be so unbearable as to make life not worth living, reducing strong and active human beings to trembling, emaciated wrecks and leading some to commit suicide. Thus, the delicate balance between excitation and inhibition in the pain system must be preserved if a normal existence is to be led.

REFERENCES

CASSINARI, V., and PAGNI, C. *Central pain.* Cambridge, Mass.: Harvard University Press, 1969, 192 pp.

CRITCHLEY, M. Congenital indifference to pain. *Annals of Internal Medicine* 45: 737–747, 1956.

NASHOLD, B.S.; URBAN, B.; and ZORUB, D.S. Phantom pain relief by focal destruction of the substantia gelatinosa of Rolando. In *Advances in Pain Research and Therapy* 1: 959–963, 1976.

WEIR MITCHELL, SILAS. *Injuries of nerves and their consequences.* Philadelphia: Lippincott, 1872, 337 pp.

9

Pain and Anesthesia

In an age when *anesthesia* has been a household word for more than a century and when every type of operation can be done painlessly, it is hard to conceive of a time when this was not so. But in that not-so-distant period, the very suggestion that pain was neither a necessary nor inevitable accompaniment of surgery would have been greeted with incredulity, derision, and sometimes with righteous indignation. Pain was something that the gods had decreed for the good of humanity; it was to be borne with fortitude and resignation; indeed, some surgeons believed that it was actually beneficial to the patient!

Lest we take anesthesia too readily for granted, it is both sobering and instructive to turn the clock back a century and a half and learn from eyewitness accounts as reported in the *Lancet,* a foremost English medical journal, what operations were actually like in that period.

It is the winter of 1836 as we visit the North-London Hospital, England, renowned for its staff of distinguished physicians and surgeons. The grim, gray building, with its dark corridors and jostling throng of humanity, bears little resemblance to its modern counterparts. On this particular day, Saturday, 27th of February, there is an air of excitement in the surgical wing, for word is about that Mr. Robert Liston, the famous surgeon, is scheduled to perform an unusual and difficult procedure. The surgery today is to take place in the operating theater, a peculiarly fitting description for the room in which the morning's events are to transpire. One wall of the high-ceilinged and forbidding room is formed almost completely by a great glass window, which allows as much illumination as possible, while several gas jets cast a fitful glow on the darker corners of the chamber.

In the center of the room stands a solid wooden operating table, from which hang a number of heavy leather restraint straps. An unruly crowd of medical students, orderlies, and assorted onlookers has assembled, vying for the best position to view the forthcoming spectacle. Dressed in their street clothes, they shove and jostle and curse each other; a fight momentarily flares up and dies down. This clamorous scene is briefly interrupted as two stalwart orderlies enter with the patient, twenty-one-year-old Ann Struther. Pale and haggard, she is helped onto the table and firmly strapped down. A prominent bulge on her left cheek partly disfigures her otherwise attractive features.

Four years previously, she had been much troubled by pain in the left side of her head and face, which was followed by swelling of the upper gum. Three teeth were extracted without providing relief, and when the swelling increased, it was excised. Despite this it returned, and two years earlier she had submitted to "a very severe operation." It too had failed to arrest the progression of the mass, which was now "as large as a moderate sized coconut." If allowed to follow its natural course, it would not only force her eye from its socket but subject her to progressive, unrelenting pain and, ultimately, cause her death. There was no alternative but to operate while there was still time.

A sudden hush falls on the assembled crowd as Liston (Figure 9.1), a commanding man of forty, strides briskly into the theater and, after transferring a gold watch and fob from his waistcoat to a trouser pocket, flings his jacket to an orderly, rolls up his sleeves, and, approaching the young woman, murmurs a few reassuring words. Then, as the orderlies immobilize her shoulders and head, with rapid, dexterous strokes of his scalpel, he cuts down to the bone, and using a forceps in preference to either the saw or the chisel to try to reduce the pain as much as possible, he severs the bony attachments and removes her left upper jaw in a single piece. The entire procedure is completed in the incredibly brief time of six minutes, despite the convulsive writhing and screaming of the unfortunate patient. Reference to Figure 4.2, which illustrates a few of the branches of the major sensory nerve to the face, may provide the reader with some notion of the innervation involved; it gives no idea, however, of the vast network of arteries and veins that are present nor of the gross enlargement of blood vessels that commonly occurs with large tumors. The procedure can only be regarded as one of remarkable heroism on the part of the patient and a tour de force by the surgeon. The excised tumor, described as an osteosarcoma, was available to "any gentleman who wishes to inspect it," and "every facility will be afforded him for that purpose, should

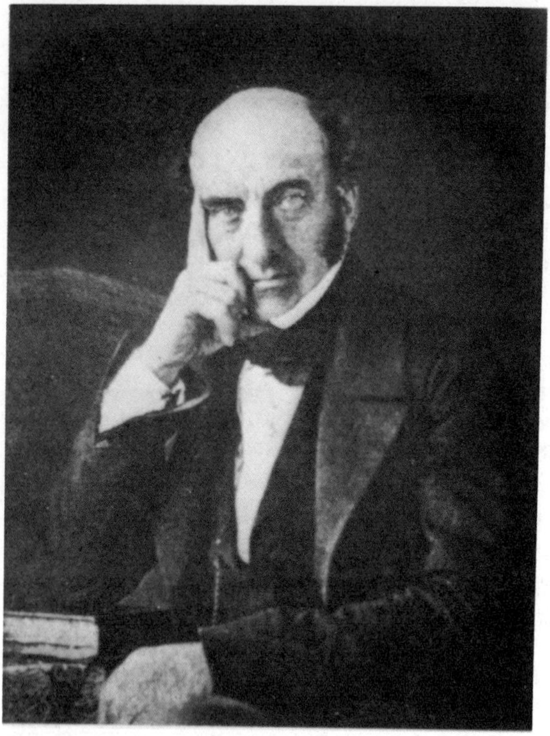

Figure 9.1. Robert Liston (1794–1847).
The son of a parish minister, Liston was born in Linlithgowshire, Scotland, and received most of his early education from his father. The parental tutoring appears to have been excellent, for the young Liston obtained a prize for Latin prose composition in 1808, shortly after entering Edinburgh University. He began his anatomical studies at age sixteen, becoming one of the outstanding surgical anatomists of his time, and was appointed house surgeon at the Royal Infirmary when he was twenty. Two years later, in 1816, Liston moved to London and received his membership in the Royal College of Surgeons, but returned to Edinburgh in 1817, remaining there until 1834. While there, he developed his unparalleled skills as a surgeon; however, his uncompromising attitude, coupled with a rough manner verging on rudeness, provoked the hostility of many of his associates and led to his expulsion from the Royal Infirmary in 1822. This action was rescinded in 1827, but when Syme was selected as Professor of Surgery (1834) in preference to him, Liston accepted the Professorship at London Hospital in 1835. He was elected to the Fellowship of the Royal Society in 1841.
Illustration courtesy of Longman Group Ltd.

he pay a visit to the hospital." Four days later, the patient was said to be doing exceedingly well.

In the same volume of the *Lancet* in which the foregoing operation is documented, there is a detailed record of an almost identical procedure carried out for removal of a large malignant tumor of the face at the Westminster Hospital by Mr. Guthrie, a surgeon of considerable repute at the time. In this instance, however, the operation lasted for forty-five minutes. The patient, one Mary Brown, a forty-six-year-old married nurse, showed almost unbelievable fortitude throughout the entire frightful procedure. As noted in the report, which describes the gruesome events in detail, "it [the operation] was borne with noble courage. Not an exclamation of pain escaped her." There follows a description of the requests by the surgeon for various instruments (scalpel, hooks, scissors, and so on), all of which as well as the clanking of instruments and exclamations and other noises were fully audible to the patient, and then the surgeon's efforts to reassure the patient, among which were: "You bear it very well, my dear lady"; "By the blessing of God, my dear soul, it is nearly over"; "Give her a little wine"; and so on. The patient slept for two hours after the operation and on succeeding days took nourishment with little trouble; three days later the wound was said to be healing satisfactorily.

Other examples of surgical procedures and related events carried out under these barbarous conditions are the following:

On one occasion Liston was about to begin an operation when, not surprisingly, the patient's courage deserted him. The unfortunate man made a dash for the door and, gaining it before he could be stopped, rushed screaming down the corridor and locked himself in a room. Liston, a large and powerful man, not the least nonplussed by this turn of events, pursued the terrified man and, after kicking the door open, dragged him back to the operating room where, with the help of his assistants, he securely strapped him down and carried out the operation as planned (see Howell 1926).

A Mr. Earle, a surgeon at St. Bartholomew's Hospital in London, was called to remove a nail from the ear of a seven-year-old boy. As reported in the *Lancet,* a probe was passed about an inch into the ear and "could be distinctly heard to strike some metallic object which appeared to be firmly impacted into the tympanum"! After a series of unsuccessful attempts to remove the "foreign object" with several pairs of forceps, the procedure was temporarily abandoned. Six days later, with the boy now in apparently good condition, the attack was resumed. The surgeon, using great force, first bent a metal probe in the child's ear canal and then, having grasped what he thought was the nail head, pulled so violently that he bent the forceps! This frightful and fruitless procedure, since no nail was recovered, lasted altogether an hour, during which time additional instruments were bent. Needless to say, the child was described as "nearly exhausted" at the end of the procedure, and he succumbed some days afterward. The ultimate tragedy is that at autopsy, no sign of a nail could be found, though the bone was markedly damaged! We must remember that neither X rays nor endoscopic instruments were available at the time to aid in the localization of a foreign body; but the dreadful suffering inflicted and the fatal outcome are in stark contrast to current expectations and results!

The scene in each instance is so bizarre by present-day standards as to test one's credulity. But such events—and no doubt others more gruesome by far that, for the sake of propriety, were never reported—occurred on a daily basis in hospitals around the world. We should remember, too, that the centers referred to were among the foremost of the period. It should not astonish us that spectators and surgeons of the period walked into operating rooms in their street clothes and boots. For no one then had the remotest idea of what caused infections; another generation was to pass before Pasteur proved conclusively that invisible organisms were responsible and before Lister, promptly grasping the enormous significance of these inspired laboratory discoveries, applied them with signal success to the control of surgical infections.

Almost unbelievably, operations on virtually every organ were performed without anesthesia by surgeons who were not or could not be deterred by the appalling suffering of their patients. Breasts were removed for cancer, arms and legs were amputated, caesarean births were frequent, and tumors of the testes, ovaries, rectum, and other organs were routinely removed. The only area that remained sacrosanct was the central nervous system, for in the few instances when a surgeon had the temerity to operate on the brain, overwhelming infection almost invariably carried off those few patients who miraculously survived the hazards of hemorrhage and trauma. Not surprisingly, even the boldest surgeons declined to do more than trephine the skull (remove a disk of bone), and that only on rare occasions.

The only way to deal with the agonizing pain of operations was to ply the patients with wine, rum, and opium and to make the experience as brief as possible; surgeons who were renowned for their dexterity and swiftness were naturally in great demand. The speed with which some of the more gifted surgeons of the period could complete an operation was legendary. Liston, for example, could amputate through the thigh and have a leg off in half a minute, but the removal of the upper jaw in six minutes, as described earlier, is if anything more astonishing. Sir Astley Cooper removed stones from the bladder in less than a minute, and the famous Syme of Edinburgh took about a minute to amputate through the hip!*

*See also Chapter 1, in which Baron Larrey's remarkable surgical skill is noted.

Bleeding was often controlled by application of the cautery, and one can only hope that by the time this stage was reached, most patients were too far gone from loss of blood and shock to feel the additional agony.

GENERAL ANESTHESIA

The idea that insensibility might be induced in order to abolish the pain of operations is an ancient one. Keys (1963) has reviewed the story from its beginnings in his scholarly *History of Surgical Anesthesia,* from which a few highlights are quoted.

The Greek god Aesculapius was said to have rendered his patients insensible during operations by administering a potion of undescribed nature named nepenthe, whereas the root of the plant mandragora was one of the favored ingredients of the concoctions used from antiquity through the Middle Ages.

Perhaps the closest approach to modern general anesthesia was achieved in the sixteenth century by Paracelsus, who—searching for an anesthetic agent—discovered sweet vitriol, now known as ether. As Keys points out, Paracelsus described how chickens were rendered insensible by its vapors but promptly regained consciousness as the effect wore off and appeared none the worse for their experience. Why ether was not introduced at that time as an anesthetic agent is not clear. Some three hundred years were to pass before the remarkable anesthetic properties of this agent were recognized and widely applied for the suppression of pain. There is no way to measure the cumulative suffering that might have been avoided by the timely introduction of this great drug.

In 1799 Sir Humphry Davy, the distinguished chemist, had proposed that nitrous oxide be used as an anesthetic, but even though the suggestion came from a man of his eminence, it was ignored.

As with many great discoveries, there are many contenders for the honor of being the founder of surgical anesthesia. It is generally agreed, however, that the first convincing public demonstration of surgical anesthesia for a major operation was given by William T. G. Morton on Friday, October 16, 1846, in Dr. John C. Warren's operating room at the Massachusetts General Hospital in Boston. Morton (Figure 9.2) administered sulfuric ether to a young man for the removal of a tumor of the jaw; on recovering consciousness, the patient stated that he had felt no pain at any time.

This spectacular demonstration fired the imagination of most physicians, and despite the relative slowness with which news traveled in those days, on December 19th of the same year, Robert Liston of London employed ether anesthesia on two patients. Initially skeptical about the method, he was startled at the end of an amputation on one patient to hear him ask: "When are you going to begin?" and then, "Take me back, I can't have it done." Liston's terse comment was, "This Yankee dodge, gentlemen, beats mesmerism hollow."

Whereas Liston and many others accepted anesthesia with enthusiasm and alacrity, others were either slow to employ it or expressed active opposition. Thus, the more conservative clergy and some physicians strongly objected to its use in childbirth on the grounds that pain was a normal phenomenon and, as such, should be borne with courage and fortitude. Such retrogressive and sadistic opinions had been voiced in an earlier period, when hypnosis was advocated for the control of pain during operations (see Chapter 13). However, the matter was summarily settled in favor of anesthesia when Queen Victoria elected to have ether for her own delivery.

In the light of what surgery meant to patients before the discovery of general anesthesia, as described in the foregoing paragraphs, it is no exaggeration to say that in every city a monument should be erected to Morton and possibly to the other pioneers who delivered humanity from the curse of operative pain. Instead, we have monuments and memorials to generals and politicians whose actions so frequently led to the frightful battlefield injuries that necessitated surgery in the first place.

What Is Anesthesia?

The word *anesthesia* was first proposed by Oliver Wendell Holmes in a letter dated November 21, 1846, to W. T. G. Morton, the pioneer of anesthesiology discussed earlier. The term means "without sensation" and was universally accepted for all agents that produce a state of insensibility.

Anesthetics that, in addition to loss of sensation, produce loss of consciousness are called *general anesthetics;* of these, the best known are ether, nitrous oxide, and pentobarbital or Pentothal; some, such as chloroform, are no longer used because of their undesirable side effects.

The gaseous general anesthetics, nitrous oxide and ether, used to be administered by means of a mask, but with advances in technique, a flexible tube is introduced into the trachea that not only allows direct access to the lungs, where the agent is absorbed, but also provides an excellent means of administering controlled respiration.

Despite the fact that general anesthetics have been known for almost 150 years, the manner in which they produce insensibility and unconsciousness has not yet been established. It is believed, because they are all highly fat-soluble substances, that they produce a reversible change in the largely fatty surface membrane of nerve cells. In a sense, the anesthetics can be regarded as toxins that damage brain cells just enough for them to

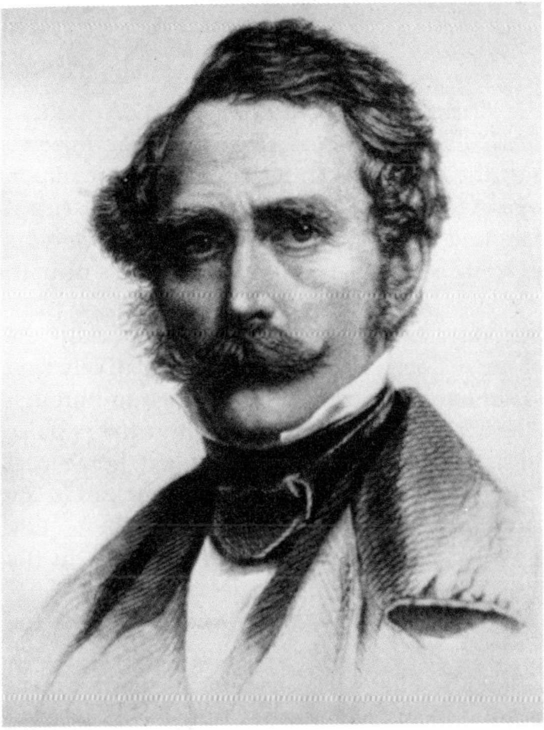

Figure 9.2 William T.G. Morton (1819–1868).
Morton, born in Charlton, Massachusetts, the son of a farmer of Scottish ancestry, entered the Baltimore College of Dentistry and was graduated in 1842. Concerned about the superficiality of his medical knowledge, he studied medicine at Harvard, but financial difficulties prevented him from receiving his doctorate.

Morton's introduction to the anesthetic properties of ether came by way of Charles Jackson, who demonstrated to the classes he taught that sulfuric ether caused loss of consciousness in animals. At the time, Morton was attempting to fit patients with artificial teeth, for which purpose he had to extract the remainder of the teeth and their roots from the jaw, an exceedingly painful procedure that few could tolerate. Encouraged by Jackson's demonstrations, Morton proceeded to anesthetize a variety of animals with ether without their showing any evidence of ill effects in recovering. Application of the method to humans was precipitated by a patient who arrived in his office on September 30, 1846, suffering great pain from toothache. Morton had him breathe the vapors of ether and then extracted the tooth without the patient's being aware that anything had happened.

Subsequent to the demonstrations at the Massachusetts General Hospital, considerable controversy developed with regard to the priority of this major discovery. Morton had also hoped to receive some financial compensation, but despite continued efforts by both him and his supporters, he was unsuccessful and lived the last years of his life in poverty.

Illustration from *The Battle for Oblivion* by Betty MacQuitty. Courtesy of Betty MacQuitty.

become transitorily inactive. Fortunately, general anesthetics have enough selectivity that only certain nerve cell populations are affected by them at a dosage that is well tolerated by other neurons, such as those that maintain and regulate respiration. These continue to function quite adequately during the anesthetic state, but they too fail if the dose of drug is increased.

Local Anesthetics

Another group of anesthetic drugs produces loss of sensation without interfering with consciousness. These, the local anesthetics, are injected either into the tissues or into the nerve trunks supplying the area upon which it is necessary to operate. A special group of these, the spinal anesthetics, can be injected around the spinal cord and/or the nerve roots that carry noxious messages to it (see Figure 5.1), producing loss of both sensation and motor power.

The local anesthetics produce their effects by interfering with the function of the membrane of nerve fibers; how this occurs is relatively well known and, in brief, consists in impairing the passage of sodium through the membrane. As a result, the nerve cannot generate a conducted impulse (described in Chapter 2), and thus signaling is brought to a halt. Some local anesthetics are applied directly to the surface of mucous membranes of the mouth, nose, trachea, or bladder, for example; they penetrate these quite readily and act on the fine, superficially distributed nerve fibers in the manner already described; these are called topical anesthetics.

The large selection of anesthetic agents that are now available and the detailed knowledge of their effects, indications, and contraindications not only makes surgery painless but also allows the surgeon to work far more effectively. In fact, the revolution in surgical practice they have caused is of incalculable value, both in terms of relief of suffering and in the opening up of entirely new fields of surgery that would otherwise have been quite impossible.

Nerve Blocks

Injection of a small amount of local anesthetic (procaine, Xylocaine, lidocaine) into or around a nerve is a valuable and widely employed method in diagnosis and treatment of painful conditions. Diagnostically, it can help to establish which nerve or dorsal root is primarily or solely responsible for pain, especially in complicated situations. It may be necessary to repeat the diagnostic nerve block several times in some instances, where the result is not clear-cut and particularly when a neurotomy or rhizotomy is being considered.

Nerve blocks can also be of particular value in providing anesthesia for surgical procedures on the limbs when a general anesthetic is considered inadvisable.

Another useful aspect of these blocks is that they give a patient an excellent idea of what to expect in terms of sensory loss when a nerve is to be transected for pain relief.

From the standpoint of treatment, anesthetic nerve blocks can be very useful if employed early in the course of a pain problem that is showing signs of becoming chronic. Sometimes a single injection or, more often, several nerve blocks given on successive days give permanent relief of pain. Precisely how this occurs is not known, though it is speculated that the sudden decrease or cessation of noxious input may somehow interrupt abnormal activity in central neuronal circuits.

Finally, nerves can be blocked for a longer time by injection of very small amounts of alcohol or phenol.

Another commonly employed variety of local anesthesia is injection into the lumbar spinal fluid or around the dura (epidural). Many surgical procedures are done in this manner; excellent anesthesia is obtained without loss of consciousness in the patient.

REFERENCES

BONICA, J.J. *The management of pain.* Philadelphia: Lea & Febiger, 1953.

HOWELL, W.B. Concerning some old medical journals. *Annals of Medical History* 8: 155–175, 1926.

KEYS, T.E. *The history of surgical anesthesia.* New York: Dover, 1963, 200 pp.

NORTH-LONDON HOSPITAL. Osteo-sarcoma of the jaw—Removal of the superior maxillary and malar bones. *Lancet* 1: 917–918, 1836.

WESTMINSTER HOSPITAL. Removal of a large malignant tumour of the cheek with a portion of the bones of the face. *Lancet* 1: 189–191, 1835.

10

Drugs in the Treatment of Pain

The quest for analgesic drugs, or painkillers, as they are frequently called in today's dramatized vocabulary, began in a long-lost past. In the *Ebers Papyrus,* an Egyptian scribe of the eighteenth dynasty (1000 B.C.,) tells of an elixir that deadened pain. We have no reason to doubt this ancient claim, for the scribe was a careful man who listed the ingredients of the remedy; one of them, as will be noted later, is employed in a purified form with signal success to this day. Whether the prescription was new at the time of writing or had long been in use, we do not know. We can safely assume, however, that it was not the first preparation tried for the relief of pain and that millennia of fruitless searching had elapsed before an effective drug was found.

Progress in analgesic medication, however, continued to be desperately slow. In the three thousand years between the day of the Egyptian scribe and the development of modern pharmacology in the nineteenth century, only one analgesic drug of real value, aspirin, was added to the pharmacopoeia.

Even with all the resources of current scientific technology, however, the ideal analgesic has yet to be developed. Such a drug should be able to be taken by mouth rather than by injection; it should act rapidly and suppress pain completely; the effect should be of adequate duration; and there should be no disagreeable or toxic side effects. These may seem to be entirely unrealistic expectations, but the same might have been said a century ago for a drug to control bacterial infections.

Paul Ehrlich (1854–1915) believed that a "magic bullet" could be found that would selectively destroy the spirochete of syphilis without injuring the host's tissues. Indefatigable workers, he and his assistants found a compound of arsenic that came close to realizing his dream on the 606th try, and the 914th was better. So, for a quarter of a century, patients were treated with Ehrlich's magic bullet, number 914 or neosalvarsan. But neo-salvarsan was toxic and did not kill all the spirochetes, especially those that had found their way into the brain; patients continued to become demented and to die, slowly, over a few years.

Ehrlich was, unfortunately, not around to see the realization of his dream. For when penicillin appeared, it did exactly what he had predicted: the spirochetes—all the spirochetes, including those in the brain—were destroyed. Yet with the sole exception of occasional allergic reactions, the drug was completely harmless to the patients' tissues.

To hope for a similar magic bullet to control pain may not be too unrealistic. Indeed, with recent striking advances in our knowledge of the biochemistry of pain pathways, it seems possible, or even probable, that the goal is within reach.

What of the analgesics that are currently available? How good are they, and what problems do they present? Basically, drugs for treatment of pain can be divided into analgesics and tranquilizers; the former deal with the pain itself, whereas the latter relieve the anguish and fear associated with chronic pain. The analgesics have classically been divided into a weak group—as exemplified by aspirin and other nonnarcotic drugs—and a strong category that includes the narcotics and certain synthetic drugs, both of which, unfortunately, have pronounced addictive potential. However, a new generation of nonnarcotic and apparently nonaddictive drugs may lead to this classification's being revised in the near future.

ASPIRIN AND OTHER WEAK ANALGESICS

Of all the drugs available for the treatment of pain, none is superior to aspirin when all factors are taken into account. This may come as a surprise to many; one tends to assume that there must be a number of drugs with fancy chemical names that are much more effective in relieving pain than humble aspirin. Surely, a drug that can be purchased over the counter without a prescription and that is available in virtually any part of the world cannot be all that good. Yet when we look at the record carefully and compare aspirin with all other painkillers, the conclusion is inescapable—aspirin is an unrivaled analgesic for mild to moderate pain. Strong analgesic drugs such as the narcotics are, of course, effective for severe pains that aspirin cannot relieve, but the grave risk of addiction limits their usefulness to pain of brief duration, such as that of the postoperative period or of acute injuries.

The origin of aspirin has been traced back into antiquity; thus, the ancients brewed a potion from willow bark that reduced patients' high fever. But it was not until 1827, when Leroux, a French chemist, isolated from the bark a substance that he called salicin, from the scientific name of the tree *(Salix alba),* that the active principle was identified. Since then, the term *salicylates* has been used to designate a group of drugs of similar composition to salicin, which have been and still are of enormous value in the treatment of pain and inflammation. The best known of these is aspirin, or acetyl salicylic acid; the others are sodium salicylate; methyl salicylate or oil of wintergreen, used in liniments for massaging aching muscles; and salicylic acid, a component of certain skin ointments.

From a practical point of view, aspirin is in many respects a remarkable drug; easy to synthesize and thus inexpensive, it produces few toxic effects if taken in moderation; and not only is it an analgesic, but it also lowers the temperature and reduces inflammation.

How Does It Work? In the past ten years or so, investigators have begun to clarify the mechanisms through which aspirin works to relieve pain. Currently it appears that one of its main actions is to depress the synthesis of prostaglandins, substances that are widely distributed in the body; it also has significant anticoagulant effects by impairing the aggregation of blood platelets.

When prostaglandins are released in the tissues as a result of inflammation or injury, they sensitize the nerve endings that relay pain signals. Aspirin inhibits the enzyme, prostaglandin synthetase, whereupon the production of prostaglandins is arrested, and the hyperexcitable nerve endings return to their normal state. In addition, aspirin lowers the temperature in cases of fever, but interestingly, it does not affect normal temperature. This antipyretic effect is also believed to be due to its inhibitory action on prostaglandins released in the hypothalamus in patients with fever. Though at one time this was regarded as an important property of the drug, it is much less prized nowadays, since the contemporary physician is usually able to treat the cause of fevers—often bacterial—with antibiotics or other specific remedies instead of combating this sign of disordered function.

How Good an Analgesic Is Aspirin? When tested by the usual laboratory methods (electric or thermal) on normal skin, no change in threshold can be detected. However, when sensitization of the skin is produced by prior injection of a chemical irritant, aspirin almost completely reverses the overreaction; that is, it is almost 100 percent effective. The reason for this is quite obvious in view of the preceding description of its mechanism of action on prostaglandin synthesis.

Weak analgesic drugs are used specifically to alleviate pain that is present for hours, days, or months. Such chronic pain is never of very high sensory intensity; on a scale of 1 to 10 (from mildest to maximum pain), it lies somewhere in the lower to mid part of the scale. This is easy to understand, for maximum pain cannot be endured for more than a second, and pain intensities between 9 and 5 on the scale are tolerated for only slightly longer periods. Of the drugs in this group, aspirin is very effective for low-intensity pains, something that everyone who has had a headache is well aware of, and especially when an inflammatory basis is present. On the other hand, more severe pain is not relieved, and increasing the dose has no further effect on pain.

Dangers of Aspirin. In view of the fact that the annual consumption of aspirin in the United States is approximately 15,000 tons, the number of unfavorable reactions to it is vanishingly small, making it one of the safest medicines available today. However, even aspirin, if taken in excessive amounts, can have serious toxic effects; parenthetically, so can any substance, including water.

If the correct dose (one or two 325-mg tablets repeated at intervals up to a total of twelve tablets a day for an adult) is taken, the great majority of people suffer no side effects. Some may have a mild degree of nausea, heartburn, or even vomiting. Very rarely, bleeding from the stomach may occur. About 2 in 1,000 people are unusually sensitive and may develop hives or an attack of asthma. On the other hand, large doses of aspirin will naturally exaggerate all these toxic effects. Excessive intake of aspirin can lead to high-tone hearing loss and to ringing in the ears (tinnitus); these symptoms usually disappear spontaneously but on occasion are persistent.

How Does Aspirin Compare with Other Analgesic Preparations? A large number of preparations for the relief of headache and other minor pains are marketed on an over-the-counter basis. The components usually include aspirin and/or one of the other weak analgesic drugs. Table 10.1 lists some of the more commonly used analgesics, including several that require a prescription because of the risk of addiction.

A question that is frequently asked is, "How much better are the various drug combinations than aspirin alone?" The answer to this question is quite unequivocal: *Aspirin alone is clearly superior to any of the analgesic combinations.* At first glance, this may seem an excessively categorical statement, especially in view of the widespread claims for greater effectiveness, greater speed, and/or fewer side effects that are widely proclaimed. However, such advertising has hopelessly confused the public

Table 10.1 COMPOSITION OF SOME OF THE MOST COMMONLY USED ORAL ANALGESICS

PROPRIETARY NAME	COMPOSITION	CONTENT IN MILLIGRAMS
Alka Seltzer	Aspirin	324
	Sodium Bicarbonate	
	Citric Acid	
Anacin	Aspirin	400
	Caffeine	32
Aspirin	Aspirin	325
Bufferin	Aspirin	487.5
	Antacids[a]	
Cope	Aspirin	421
	Methapyrilene	12.5
	Caffeine	32
	Antacids[a]	
Darvon[b]	Propoxyphene	65
Detril	Acetaminophen	487.5
Empirin Compound	Aspirin	227
	Phenacetin	162
	Caffeine	32
Excedrin	Aspirin	195
	Acetaminophen	162.5
	Salicylamide	130
	Methapyrilene	25
Fiorinal[b]	Aspirin	200
	Butalbital	50
	Phenacetin	130
	Caffeine	40
Ponstel[c]	Mefenamic Acid	250
Talwin[b]	Pentazocine	30 or 60
Tylenol	Acetaminophen	300
Vanquish	Aspirin	227
	Acetaminophen	194
	Caffeine and Antacids[a]	33

[a] Antacids are usually aluminum and magnesium hydroxide.
[b] Indicates potential for addiction; prescription required.
[c] Ponstel requires a prescription, although no addictive potential is known.

and contributed significantly to clouding the basic issues. It is not surprising that this should have occurred, since the profits to be gleaned from an annual market estimated in the neighborhood of $1 billion are not inconsiderable!

The question of comparison of aspirin with other analgesic preparations can be broken down into four separate topics, which are (1) the comparative potency of aspirin versus other weak analgesics, (2) combinations of drugs versus aspirin alone, (3) the question of advantages from the addition of antacids to aspirin tablets, and (4) comparative cost.

1. With respect to the first question, the two drugs to be considered are phenacetin and acetaminophen. It has been known for many years that both drugs have approximately the same analgesic potency as aspirin, but neither of them has the antiinflammatory properties of aspirin; thus aspirin continues to be the drug of choice in most instances.
2. Most of the name-brand analgesics sold over the counter contain aspirin, together with either phenacetin, acetaminophen, or caffeine or more than one of these ingredients.

   Because of the claims made for these medications, a careful double-blind study (i.e., neither the patients nor the physicians knew what medication was being taken) was carried out at the Mayo Clinic by Moertel and his colleagues (1974) to try to settle the issue in a responsible and definitive manner. One hundred patients with mild to moderate pain due to inoperable cancer were selected for the study. All patients were ambulant and were judged to be intelligent and capable observers. The chart (Figure 10.1) summarizes results of their study and is worthy of careful perusal. First, it shows what many others have found—that a placebo, in this case, a sugar (lactose), has a definitely perceptible effect, for 20 percent of patients claimed to detect significant (more than 50 percent) relief of their pain.

   Next, aspirin alone had a clearly superior effect to the placebo, since 40 percent of patients reported significant relief of pain. Particularly interesting is the fact that the addition of caffeine, of sedatives (pentobarbital), tranquilizers (chlorpromazine), or another mild analgesic (ethoheptazine or propoxyphene, known as Darvon) results in no improvement whatsoever over the analgesia produced by asprin alone. To quote their comment verbatim:

> Thirty-two milligrams of caffeine plus 400 mg of aspirin is the Anacin formula. Over-the-counter products such as Excedrin, Vanquish, Empirin Compound and APC compounds (i.e., aspirin, phenacetin, caffeine), are mixtures of caffeine plus a lesser dose of aspirin (195–227 mg) with the deficit in aspirin made up by the addition of other analgesic–antipyretics such as phenacetin, acetaminophen or salicylamide. Although each of these preparations is several times as expensive as generic aspirin, *there is no acceptable evidence that any provides the patient with more effective pain therapy."* [Emphasis added]

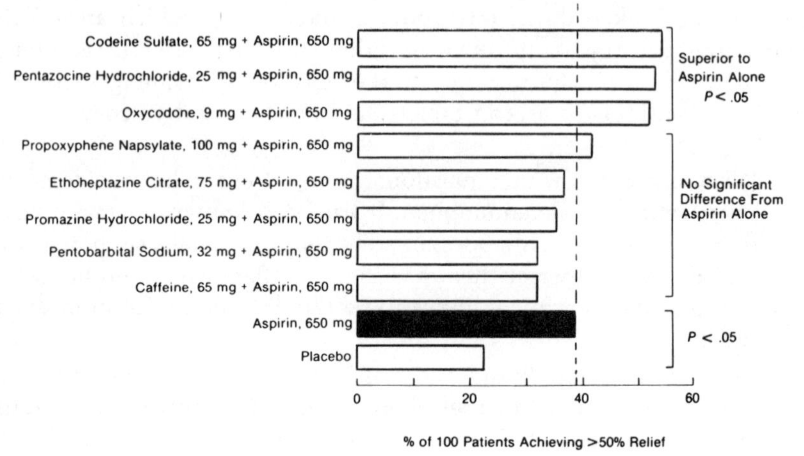

Comparative therapeutic effect of placebo, aspirin alone, and aspirin combinations according to percentage of patients achieving significant (ie, more than 50%) relief of pain.

Figure 10.1. At the Mayo Clinic, the efficacy of a series of commonly prescribed analgesics was evaluated in patients with chronic pain. As this graph shows, aspirin alone is better than combinations of drugs; it was surpassed only when narcotics were added.

Reprinted by permission of the *Journal of the American Medical Association* 229: 55–59, 1974; and the authors, Charles G. Moertel et al. © 1974, American Medical Association.

The addition of sedatives or tranquilizers to aspirin, with the intent of diminishing the anxiety and apprehension that are so commonly associated with chronic pain, not only failed in its objective of potentiating aspirin but was decried by the investigators because of the risk of addiction associated with this group of drugs.

A large proportion of analgesic drug combinations are not only inferior to aspirin but actually irrational. This statement is not in any way an attempt at sensationalism, but is the opinion stated in the *AMA Drug Evaluations Handbook* as far back as the first edition in 1971. This authoritative survey by a committee of thirteen experts on drug actions and effects lists no less than ninety-three brand-name analgesic mixtures that are described either as irrational, not recommended, or both.

In summary, there is no brand-name drug or combination of drugs currently available on a nonprescription basis (this eliminates those that contain narcotics) that is any more effective, by any measure, or that has fewer side effects or any other demonstrable advantage when compared to plain aspirin.

Another claim that is sometimes made is that certain combinations of aspirin with other drugs result in much faster pain relief.

Although it is true that the absorption rate of aspirin can be increased or decreased to a considerable degree, it is unlikely that the differences(s) would be detected. Even if it were, how many headaches or other minor pains (the only pains for which aspirin is appropriate) require such fast relief? If the headache is relieved in seven minutes instead of eight or nine, the difference seems too trivial to be noticeable or even worthy of comment.

The inescapable conclusion is that aspirin alone is the drug of choice for the relief of minor pains such as headache, rheumatism, muscular pains, toothache, and bursitis.

Combinations of aspirin with codeine or derivatives of codeine, such as oxymorphone, or with pentazocine were found by Moertel et al. to be significantly more effective than aspirin alone in relieving pain. However, it hardly needs to be pointed out that these additional ingredients are narcotics, whose analgesic properties are already greater than those of aspirin.

Of course, the use of a narcotic in combination with several other ingredients of somewhat dubious credentials has been a standby for quite some time. Take, for example, the following prescription for headache:

Berry of the Coriander 1	Berry of the Sames plant 1
Berry of the Poppy plant 1	Berry of the Juniper plant 1
Wormwood 1	Honey 1

Make into one, mix with honey, and simmer therewith in order to make him well forthwith. When the remedy is used by him against all illnesses of the head and all sufferings and evils of any sort, he will instantly become well. [*Papyrus Ebers,* quoted in Bryan 1974]

This prescription was used successfully more than three thousand years ago by the woman doctor Isis to cure the Great Ra of an intractable headache. The caption reads: "Another remedy which the goddess Isis prepared for the god Ra to drive out the pains that are in his head." Of course, the active ingredient was opium contained in the berry of the poppy plant, and perhaps the prescription was as efficient as some of the better ones available today!

3. Aspirin not infrequently produces some degree of heartburn or mild nausea in susceptible people. The addition of antacids seems to be a perfectly reasonable response to this minor side effect. However, a panel of the National Academy of Sciences that studied the problem concluded that there was no evidence whatsoever to indicate that buffered aspirin compounds were any less irritant to the stomach

than plain aspirin. Larger amounts of antacids would probably reduce stomach upsets, but the same result can be obtained by taking the drug with a large glass of water or milk.

4. From the standpoint of economy, aspirin is incomparably the better buy. Some of the brand-name products may cost up to eighteen times the price of a therapeutically equivalent amount of plain aspirin of a perfectly acceptable brand! This statement is based on inquiries at several local pharmacies; the lowest price quoted for 100 tablets of plain aspirin was $0.59, and the highest was $10.50 for 100 tablets of a combination rated "irrational" by the *AMA Drug Evaluation Handbook.* Yet according to *Consumers Reports* (1972), brand-name products consume four fifths of every dollar spent on over-the-counter analgesics, with aspirin accounting for only one fifth. Such is the power of advertising!

There are certain infrequent situations in which, as noted earlier, some people are hypersensitive to aspirin; thus, patients with asthma, bleeding tendencies, or stomach ulcers are usually unable to tolerate aspirin. In these cases another drug such as acetaminophen may be used with success; a physician should make this decision.

As an epilogue to the foregoing review of modern commercial pharmacology, Moertel's wry introduction to one of his studies (1976) on the comparative efficiency of oral analgesics can scarcely be improved upon.

> Take ye a lock of Vergins haire on any part of ye head. . . . Cut it very smale to fine powder then take 12 ants eggs dried in an oven after ye bread is drawne or other wise make them dry and make them to powder with the haire, give this with a quarter of a pint of red cow's milk or, for want of it give it in strong ale wort.
>
> Prescription for pain
> Written by Zerobabbel Endecott
> Physician at Salem, 1659

But how about its modern equivalent!

> Take ye 450 mg of Paracetamol and make it to a fine powder. Add to this 5 mg of Doxylamine to make the patient sleepy and 30 mg of Caffeine to keep him awake. Then take 9.75 mg of Codeine and make them all to fit into a multicolored capsule. When this is done, call it Mersyndol and buy a full page ad in the Medical Journal of Australia.
>
> Prescription for pain
> Written by the Wm. S. Merrell Co.,
> Sydney, 1974

The preceding comments should not be taken in any sense as a blanket indictment of drug-producing companies but only of the type of publicity engaged in by some firms, which can only be described as misleading and deceptive advertising. Balanced against this, the public should remember that most of these companies are engaged in extremely costly research that has led to the synthesis of many new drugs whose enormous benefits to humanity cannot be overemphasized. Moreover, exhaustive evaluation of every new drug in experimental animals, the highest standards of quality control, and detailed information provided to physicians by the scientific departments of these companies help to serve the patient extremely well in the vast majority of instances.

New, Potent Aspirin-Like Drugs

Aspirin, as noted earlier, inhibits the production of prostaglandins, substances that are released from within cells during inflammation, by certain insect stings and by exposure to ultraviolet light. It is, however, not the only drug that acts in this manner; among others that do, indomethacin, which was introduced almost twenty years ago, is actually some ten times as potent as aspirin, but it has a greater tendency to produce toxic side effects.

One of the most encouraging developments in recent times is the introduction of analgesic agents of this type that are far more potent than aspirin or even morphine but that nonetheless appear to be devoid of addictive potential.

Among these, zomepirac, marketed by McNeill Laboratories as Zomax, gives promise of being a major breakthrough in the treatment of chronic pain.

Codeine. Though commonly included in the group of strong analgesics, codeine ranks somewhere between aspirin and morphine. Like aspirin, it can be taken by mouth, and in a dose of 65 mg it is said to produce approximately the same analgesic effect as 650 mg of aspirin. However, in a study by Moertel et al. (1972), codeine at this dosage was inferior to aspirin; only when the dosage was increased to 120 mg was it shown to be significantly better. In certain situations codeine is preferable to aspirin —for example, when pain and cough occur together, since codeine depresses the cough reflex. However, the latter property may be a disadvantage when the cough is performing the useful function of removing excessive secretions.

Though a vast number of patients have been treated with codeine, it is extremely rare for addiction to occur; in those few who use it for psychological reasons, the degree of dependence is minor and the habit, easily broken. However, because of this minor risk of dependence, it has been placed on the list of restricted substances.

The undesirable side effects of codeine vary considerably in intensity among different people. Nausea and vomiting are quite common and often sufficiently severe to require changing to another analgesic; constipation is a usual result after repeated doses, and dizziness or drowsiness are not uncommon. All in all, the indications for taking codeine instead of aspirin are quite limited.

STRONG ANALGESICS: THE NARCOTICS

Morphine

Sir William Osler, the great physician of the turn of the century, used to call morphine "God's own medicine"; and no wonder, for at a time when there were, at most, a dozen drugs of any value at all, here was one that was potent, had many uses, and was cheap and readily available.

This remarkable drug is also one of the oldest known; there is evidence that it was known to the Sumerians six thousand years ago. It seems probable that it was used mainly for its effects on emotions, for even then its name meant "joy." The Ancient Greeks knew of it, for Homer recorded Helen of Troy's signal success with the elixir nepenthe, no doubt due to the opium it contained. Long before its analgesic qualities were known, its inhibitory action on bowel contractions was employed for victims of dysentery; cramping pains decreased and lethal dehydration was diminished. In an age when bacteria had not been dreamed of and fluid replacement was limited to what could be taken by mouth and kept down, it was as near to a panacea as humanity could come.

Morphine's analgesic properties were apparently recognized in the Middle Ages, for opium was prescribed frequently for the control of pain. Paracelsus (1493–1541) is credited with introducing laudanum, a 10 percent solution of opium in water and alcohol, which has been a standby of generations of physicians up to our day. In the seventeenth and eighteenth centuries, innumerable potions and elixirs were dreamed up that contained half a dozen or more ingredients, of which opium was a frequent and popular component. Most if not all of the others were useless, but the complexity of the formulas, which, moreover, were written in Latin with a sprinkling of ritualistic abbreviations, added greatly to the mystery of a wondrous pharmacopoeia and, most importantly, to the stature of the physician in the eyes of an uninformed public.

When, in the early years of the past century, methods were developed that made it possible to split up complex substances into their component molecules—modern analytical chemistry—it was natural that one of the first questions should be, "What is the constituent in opium that relieves pain?" The answer was soon provided by the German chemist Friedrich Wilhelm Sertürner, who in 1803 isolated the active principle and named it morphine because, among other actions, it induced somnolence (from the Greek god of dreams, Morpheus).

In addition to morphine, several other molecules that acted on animal tissue were isolated from opium; codeine is the best known and most widely used of these.

How Morphine Works. The isolation of morphine meant that the most active element of opium could now be prescribed in exact amounts and that investigators could determine its effects on tissues with far greater accuracy. However, it is quite an extraordinary fact that although almost two centuries have elapsed since chemical isolation was achieved, until very recently no one had the vaguest idea of how morphine alleviated pain. Whether it worked on peripheral nerve endings, on damaged tissues, or on pain centers in the brain was anyone's guess. And when the way it works was finally established, the explanation was not only remarkable but opened up entirely new and unexpected approaches to the control of pain.

The modern phase of this fascinating story begins in 1964 with a report by Tsou and Jang, two Chinese scientists, who showed that profound analgesia was consistently produced by injecting minute amounts of morphine into a very discrete zone in the brain. This area borders on the third ventricle, the slitlike cavity in the midline of the brain. (Subsequently it has been shown that this morphine-sensitive zone of the brain continues downward along the periaqueductal gray area.)

What was particularly striking about their finding was that less than one-thousandth of the usual subcutaneous or intravenous dose of morphine produced an equivalent degree of analgesia when injected into this area; when injected into other parts of the brain, the effect was not obtained. Their findings have been confirmed and extended subsequently in laboratories around the world.

Meanwhile, and entirely independently, several teams of pharmacologists had been approaching the problem of mechanisms of morphine analgesia in a totally different way, which, nevertheless, was to converge with the findings of the Chinese researchers.* The pharmacologists had been speculating for some years that there had to be a receptor on the nerve cells that are specifically affected by morphine. What this means is simply that if a substance is given in comparatively low dosage

*Led by Avram Goldstein (Stanford), John Hughes and H. W. Kosterlitz (Edinburgh), Solomon Snyder (Johns Hopkins), and Lars Terenius (Sweden).

and it produces a relatively marked effect on certain cells (tissues), such special affinity is due to a key-and-lock type of relationship. That is, only one key (morphine in this case) will fit the lock (receptor) on the cell's surface. Experimental proof of this hypothesis was very difficult to achieve but was finally obtained. Much more exciting than this technical triumph was the question: "Why should cells have receptors for a drug to which, under normal conditions, they are never exposed?"

The Enkephalin Story

The potential answer—of transcendental significance, as we shall see—was that an unknown substance with analgesic properties might be produced normally in the body. If this were true, a natural analgesic presumably perfectly harmless to the body might be isolated and, in due course, used in the treatment of pain. Perhaps the ideal solution to an age-old problem was at hand; possibly the "magic bullet" was soon to be found. The problem then was to devise a means to test this fascinating possibility.

The method that was used was to prepare extracts of brain and test them for morphinelike activity. Since morphine, among its numerous actions, blocks contraction produced by stimulation of smooth muscle—that is, the muscle that is found in the blood vessels, intestines, and other internal organs—the brain extracts were tested against thin strips of smooth muscle. First, Hughes and co-workers (1975) and, within a few months, Snyder and associates reported that, indeed, there was an active principle in the brain extracts that blocked the stimulated contraction of smooth muscle in a way virtually identical to the blocking elicited by morphine. Not only that but certain areas of the brain were much richer in this morphinelike substance than others, notably the periventricular gray area from which Tsou and Jang had obtained the pronounced analgesic responses with vanishingly small doses of morphine.

The new substance was named "enkephalin" by Hughes and Kosterlitz to indicate that it is an *end*ogenous, (i.e., produced in the body) substance originating in the en*kepha*lon (brain). After this, it was only a matter of months before the structure of this compound was determined; as shown by Hughes and associates, it is a short chain peptide composed of five amino acids: tyrosine–glycine–glycine–phenylalanine–methionine. When given to animals, it produces analgesia comparable to that obtained with morphine; its analgesic action can be blocked by administering naloxone, a highly specific and widely used antagonist to morphine's effects, thus further emphasizing enkephalin's similarity to the latter.

Since then, a vast amount of work has been done on enkephalin; some of the more interesting facts are that certain limited modifications of the molecule can significantly prolong its effects by delaying the action of enzymes (polypeptidases), which rapidly break down the original form. It has been claimed that it is present in above-normal amounts in the spinal fluid of patients with various types of chronic pain, and particularly significant and somewhat discouraging, there is evidence already that tolerance develops to it in much the same way that it does to morphine. Tolerance signifies that as the organism is exposed to repeated doses of a given drug, it becomes progressively less sensitive to it, either because it produces large amounts of enzymes that destroy the drug, because it becomes more effective at excreting it or combining it with other substances and thus inactivating it, because a change occurs in the sensitivity of the receptor with which the drug interacts, or because of a combination of these or other mechanisms. While these discoveries were being made, investigators found a number of other endogenously produced substances with similar analgesic properties including the group of endorphins—much more complex amino acids formed by the pituitary gland.

How Do the Enkephalins Produce Their Analgesic Effects? This also has turned out to be quite an intricate phenomenon. Although the enkephalins are stored in numerous sites in the brain, in many of which they probably play no role in pain, consideration can be limited here to those found in the periaqueductal gray area, a region that is intimately concerned with the effects of morphine on pain. When enkephalin is released, it activates nerve cells in the periaqueductal gray, which discharge impulses down their axons to activate the nucleus raphé magnus located in the midline of the medulla or lower part of the brain stem. It in turn sends impulses to the spinal cord that dampen the influx of pain-producing messages to nociceptive cells in the spinal cord. In this, we see the biochemical activity of the descending control system for pain, described from a purely physiologic point of view in Chapter 2. An important point regarding this particular descending system is that it uses serotonin as its neurotransmitter; at a later point, when the most recent advances in the biochemistry of pain are discussed, this issue is noted again.

How Good an Analgesic Is Morphine? The answer to this question is "Just about the best we have." Given in optimal dosage, its effects range from complete suppression to marked reduction in the intensity of pain. When pain control is not achieved with an appropriately determined dose of morphine, further increases in dosage have no additional influence on pain. Not only does morphine alleviate pain sensation, but it also has a beneficial influence on the emotional component, an action that is almost as important in many patients as its analgesic function. The elevation of spirits (euphoria) that it produces in a significant proportion of patients helps to make life more bearable and may result in less attention being paid to the discomfort.

These are the positive aspects of morphine, but it also has some drawbacks. As with many drugs, if morphine has to be given for extended periods of time, tolerance will develop; some degree of tolerance can be demonstrated within as little as twenty-four to forty-eight hours. Since it is a progressive phenomenon, increasing doses have to be given in cases of chronic pain. Thus, the standard dose of 10 mg of morphine given every four to six hours may be quite effective for a week or so, but it becomes gradually less potent beyond this period. Yet how often is this standard dose administered for many weeks and months to patients with pain from cancer, without any thought being given to the rapidly changing scene? Increasing tolerance and thus less effectiveness are compounded by increasing pain as the cancer progresses. This phenomenon of tolerance and how to deal with it should be one of the most important aspects of a medical student's exposure to pharmacology. Yet it is often lost sight of in a welter of esoteric details of drug actions that, though of the greatest importance to the investigator, will probably never affect the physician's actual practice of medicine.

One may well ask how great tolerance can become. In my own work on morphine in the laboratory, I found, as had others, that normal rats weighing approximately 500 gm survived doses of 40 to 60 mg of morphine, but above that level they expired if they had never been exposed to the drug before. On the other hand, if they were given frequent and gradually increasing doses of morphine over a period of a month, they readily tolerated up to 300 mg—that is, more than five times the lethal dose. But much more striking than this is the observation made over thirty years ago at the U.S. Government Center for Research on Drug Addiction at Lexington, Kentucky. At the time there was a large population of drug addicts, a number of whom were voluntarily cooperating in the investigative program. In one of the studies, it was decided to find out just how tolerant to morphine a long-term addict might be. The astonishing dose of 4,560 mg of morphine was given to one subject without any adverse effects being felt or observed. The usual dose of morphine is 10 mg, and the lethal dose for nonaddicts is estimated to be somewhere between 150 and 250 mg; certain addicts can thus tolerate some twenty times the lethal dose and perhaps considerably more. The lethal amount for addicts was, of course, not established but may indeed be much greater.

Addiction. Overshadowing all its great virtues as a pain reliever, morphine's major shortcoming is its strong propensity to induce addiction and the grave consequences that ensue. Since virtually all drugs that have potent pain-relieving properties are also strongly addictive, some comments on addiction are both interesting and necessary.

Addiction or dependence is basically a need for something that may be normal, such as the need for water or food, though we don't refer to these needs as addictions; or a craving for some originally unnecessary substance, which subsequently becomes more or less indispensable. The degree of dependence varies greatly, according to the substance, the individual, and the frequency of exposure.

Thus, some drugs are only moderately addictive, good examples being tobacco and marijuana. But this is only a generalization, since there are significant numbers of people who find it extremely difficult to break dependence on tobacco. Personal idiosyncrasies are a major factor; we all are familiar with the three- and four-pack-a-day smoker who would rather take his or her chances with cancer than relinquish cigarettes. Some of these heavy smokers are never able to give up their dependence, though they make repeated attempts. Conversely, there are smokers who are quite content with a cigarette taken after each meal; they never escalate their intake of tobacco, again for rather obscure reasons that we refer to as *idiosyncrasy,* an expression that means only personal peculiarity. Giving up smoking involves no particular sacrifice for these people.

Addiction to other drugs and, specifically, to narcotics, on the other hand, is a far more serious matter; but again, idiosyncrasy plays a significant role. Much appears to depend on the motivation for taking narcotics in the first place. Thus, it has been a common experience among neurosurgeons to find that patients who had been taking large doses of morphine for pain, on being relieved of their pain by an operation, made no further demand for the drug; surprisingly, some have few or even no signs of physical withdrawal—that is, the cramping, sweating, gooseflesh, and nausea that characterize sudden interruption of narcotic intake by an addict.

On the other hand, people who take narcotics for emotional reasons, such as insecurity, anguish, loneliness, and depression, appear to become psychically and physically dependent, possibly in direct proportion to the intensity of the emotional need that originally prompted their resort to drugs. And the more intense their dependence becomes, the more difficult it is for them to break the habit.

Addiction is a disorder or disease and not, as used to be thought by many, a moral failing or weakness of character. This can best be illustrated by the fact that virtually all animals tested to date, ranging from mice and rats to monkeys, become addicted to narcotics under laboratory conditions. In this situation there is obviously no moral issue involved. Again, among experimental animals, quite striking differences may be observed in the development of addiction. In some instances, I have had monkeys become addicted to morphine within five days to a week, whereas on rare occasions it has been quite impossible to train a monkey to take morphine, though every effort was made for a period of two to three months. Some monkeys, given free access to morphine, rapidly increase their daily intake of the drug to very high levels, whereas others seem to be quite satisfied with a third or a quarter as much. Some show intense signs of withdrawal if their drug supply is stopped whereas others are barely if at all affected.

In humans, the parallels are striking, some individuals being able to break the habit quite effortlessly, whereas others are trapped by it as in quicksand, their every effort to escape being unavailing and despair engulfing them as the hopelessness of their plight becomes ever more apparent.

The foregoing comments on addiction to narcotics may perhaps emphasize sufficiently that potent analgesic drugs have unpredictable but often very serious risks of addiction. The questions might then be asked: (1) Granted that addiction may occur and often does, apart from the withdrawal symptoms, which can be avoided by taking more of the drug, to what serious problems is the addict exposed? (2) Does prolonged use of narcotic drugs impair or in some way affect mental ability, or does it lead to disorders of other organs?

Long-term intake of narcotics has not been shown to produce any significant intellectual impairment, provided of course that the individual dosage is not high enough to impair consciousness. Many addicts function, insofar as can be detected, in an entirely normal fashion while taking a narcotic. The British system, which legally provides addicts with their narcotic requirements, is based in part upon this fact. There are several major problems that beset narcotic addicts, however: their dependence on illegal and thus extortionately expensive sources for their drug needs, the uncertainty of the purity and dosage of the drugs they acquire from such sources, and, finally, the risk of blood-borne infections such as bacterial endocarditis and hepatitis when rapid and maximal effects are sought through self-administered intravenous injections using contaminated syringes and vials.

PAIN AND ADDICTION

In view of the preceding comments, what course should be followed in treating patients with chronic pain, since the most potent painkillers are the most addictive of drugs? The answer to this must be that patients with chronic pain who have potentially normal life spans for their age should not be given narcotics, since they are liable to develop some degree of addiction. On the other hand, the argument that is occasionally expressed

—that narcotics should not be administered to a given patient because of the risk of addiction—is totally unwarranted when that patient has pain due to terminal cancer and survival may be a matter of weeks or months. What possible difference can addiction make to a person in such a position? One might also remember, as noted earlier, that patients who take narcotics to relieve pain are less likely to become addicted than those who do so for one of the several psychological reasons that have been cited.

New, Strong, "Nonaddicting" Analgesics: The Antagonist/Analgesics

These drugs are among the most exciting developments in the struggle against pain, for they appear to fulfill nearly all the requirements of the "magic bullet" concept that introduced this chapter. They derived from the ideas on interactions between morphine and receptors referred to earlier in this chapter. Morphine molecules attach in a highly specific manner to receptors in the surface membrane of cells, among which are neurons in the pain pathways. Certain drugs such as Naline, naloxone, and naltrexone produce a dramatic reversal of morphine effects by displacing the latter and binding to the receptors in a process called competitive inhibition. Theoretically, then, one would expect that these morphine antagonists might also induce analgesia, and indeed some do, though others do not. Thus, naloxone is a pure antagonist of morphine and, when administered to a subject who has had no contact with morphine, produces no detectable effects—analgesic or otherwise; that is, it appears virtually inert. On the other hand, nalorphine does produce a mild analgesia, but unpleasant side effects such as anxiety and depression make it undesirable in the treatment of pain.

The fact that some morphine antagonists have analgesic qualities and, most importantly, are apparently devoid of abuse potential immediately suggests that similar drugs might be developed that lack the disagreeable side effects but retain the analgesic potency of morphine. Intense efforts along these lines over the past decade appear to have been rewarded with success, for in 1979 several antagonists with analgesic potency comparable to morphine, but devoid of addictive properties, either were approved or are awaiting approval by the U.S. Food and Drug Administration. These are nalbuphine (trade name Nubain, Endo Laboratories), buprenorphine (Tengesic, Eaton Laboratories), butorphanol (Stadol, Bristol Laboratories), and propiram (Dirame, Schering Laboratories). One shortcoming they have in common is that they are not yet available in tablet form and must be injected. This, of course, is impractical in ambulant patients with chronic pain. However, it is anticipated that an oral form will soon be developed.

At this time, the claim that they are not habit-forming appears to be well established; in addition, they do not cause the depression of the respiratory center that is characteristic of most narcotics. Whether the absence of addiction potential will continue to be substantiated as further experience is gained with them cannot, of course, be predicted. At the moment they appear extremely promising, but a degree of caution is necessary, since virtually all potent analgesics that have been introduced with the belief that they lacked abuse potential have defrauded initial optimism.

The best example of this is heroin; introduced toward the end of the last century under the impression that it was nonaddictive, it turned out to be one of the most dangerous of all narcotics. Darvon (propoxyphene), Talwin (pentazocine), and methadone are other examples of analgesics that were initially thought to lack addictive potential.

The present generation of antagonist analgesics appears to have varying degrees of undesirable side effects (hallucinations, mild depression, or anxiety) depending on the dosage required, and this may be a limiting factor in their use for severe pain. On the other hand, a very encouraging aspect is that tolerance does not appear to develop to them, even after prolonged administration. At this time they appear to be approximating the ideal for analgesics, provided further refinements in their structure can be achieved.

TREATMENT OF ANXIETY AND DEPRESSION: THE TRANQUILIZERS

As noted on numerous occasions in this book, pain is a complex experience, the two main components of which are the perception of the stimulus in terms of its intensity and nature (cutting, burning, stinging, crushing, and so on) and the response thereto, which covers a wide gamut of emotions such as agitation, fear, apprehension, anxiety, and depression.

Analgesic drugs of the several types described in the preceding pages alleviate the perception of pain to a variable degree, but in many instances —particularly when pain is of long standing and poorly controlled by analgesic drugs—anxiety and depression are frequently associated with it. In fact, the emotional symptoms may become extremely disruptive of the patient's life-style. Furthermore, the psychologic turmoil makes it even more difficult to tolerate the background of constant pain, so that, in effect, a vicious cycle is set up whereby one aspect of the disorder sensitizes the subject to the effects of the other, and vice versa.

It is in these instances of chronic pain with a more or less pronounced depressive or anxious component in which the psychotropic drugs may be of considerable value. Currently, a large spectrum of such drugs are available; the selection of the appropriate one requires careful evaluation of the individual circumstances by a physician experienced in their actions and side effects, some of which can be serious.

What these drugs do is either increase or decrease the levels of neurotransmitters (dopamine, norepinephrine, serotonin, for example) in the central nervous system (see Chapter 2) and, in this way, modulate the activity of circuitry in the limbic and related systems concerned with emotions. Because of their potential to induce addiction, they should be used sparingly and with appropriate safeguards.

NEW APPROACHES

In the past the search for new pain-relieving drugs was, to a great extent, empirical or semiscientific. This was because nothing was known about the chemical processes that took place in the complex phenomena of pain; it was therefore difficult or impossible to predict whether a new drug might have analgesic properties and, even more so, to design drugs with this specific objective. Once analytical methods had established the composition and structure of known analgesic drugs such as morphine, the logical step was to synthesize compounds of similar structure to see whether they also were analgesics, whether they were more or less potent, and, very importantly, whether they might be free of addictive properties. This approach had only limited success: A considerable number of synthetic narcotics was developed, none of which were significantly better in this respect than morphine; and despite high hopes that they would not lead to addiction, this expectation did not materialize.

Modifying the structure of a known analgesic drug may lead to the discovery of additional drugs that act in a similar manner, but the likelihood of discovering a group of drugs with entirely new and better analgesic properties is relatively remote. The other major approach is to screen drugs in a systematic manner to try to identify any that have analgesic properties. This is a time-consuming and usually unsuccessful strategy. Finally, there is the serendipitous discovery of analgesic qualities in a drug being used for other reasons.

An entirely new attack on the problem is now developing out of our increasingly accurate knowledge of the chemical substances used by the nervous system in the transmission of messages. As noted briefly in Chapter 2, when a message has flashed along an axon, a minute amount of one of these neurotransmitters is released at its end. This leads to activation of a second neuron, and so on. Of special importance is the fact that a number of different neurotransmitters have been identified, and more are being discovered every year. For many neurotransmitters, drugs have been developed that can either increase or block their concentration at the site where they are released and thus modify their effectiveness. Since some neurotransmitters have excitatory functions whereas others have inhibitory functions, and because a given system may use two or more transmitters, the number of combinations and permutations that can be induced by judicious administration of drugs that act at the transmission point is quite considerable.

In the case of pain mechanisms, there is good evidence that substance P, a peptide composed of eleven amino acids, is the excitatory neurotransmitter used by the first axon in the pain pathway. That is, it is released by the processes of the peripheral nerves when they end in the central nervous system. It is also possible that substance P may be released at other, higher stages in the pain pathway. There is evidence, too, that other neurotransmitters, such as serotonin and norepinephrine, play important roles in altering the transmission of pain messages to the brain.

Without going into the fine detail of neurotransmitter activity in pain, a few examples will serve to indicate some of the possibilities. In 1979, a drug named capsaicin was shown specifically to destroy nerve terminals containing substance P. That same year, Yaksh et al. showed that when it was injected into the cerebrospinal fluid—a crystal-clear liquid that surrounds the spinal cord (and brain)—at least half the animals so treated lost their responses to painful stimulation of the skin. What was especially important about this finding was that the effect was long-lasting and there was no evidence of impairment of other functions such as touch, motor power, or reflexes.

In other words, it appeared that the pain pathway could be destroyed in a highly selective and enduring manner by the simple expedient of injecting a drug by spinal puncture. The obvious potential for using capsaicin in the treatment of patients suffering from chronic, unbearable pain, such as that resulting from cancer, can well be imagined. Certainly, further experimental studies will have to be carried out to ensure that there are no serious side effects, but the results to date are remarkably encouraging.

Another experimental approach to the control of pain, also developed by Yaksh (Yaksh and Wilson 1979), is based on the knowledge that release of the neurotransmitter serotonin in the spinal cord has an inhibitory effect on the transmission of pain signals. Serotonin levels can be increased by administration of a drug that inhibits the breakdown of this transmitter. When pain thresholds were tested in animals so treated, it was found that they were significantly elevated.

In each of the foregoing instances, barring some quite remarkable coincidence, discovery of these pharmacological methods of controlling pain by the conventional approaches of past years would have been virtually impossible. The importance of basic research that, in its initial stages, appears to have no bearing on the practical problems of treating disease is strikingly highlighted by these advances. Thus, when Otto Loewi identified the first neurotransmitter more than half a century ago, there was no reason to suspect that it might have any bearing on pain mechanisms; and, of course, it did not in a direct fashion, since the neurotransmitter was acetylcholine, which is released mainly by nerve terminals that control motor activity. But the experiments laid the basis for the enormous edifice of neurotransmitter physiology and pharmacolgy that is essential to the understanding of how the brain works and, as a logical extension, to a deeper knowledge of the mechanisms of pain.

Where this newly acquired knowledge will lead over the coming years is difficult to predict. It seems safe to assume, however, that better and more effective methods of controlling pain will be developed as we obtain greater insight into the enormously complex neural networks whose activity spells pain, anguish, and suffering.

REFERENCES

AMA Drug Evaluations. AMA Council on Drugs, American Medical Association, Chicago, Ill., 1971.

BRYAN, C.P. Translation of German version of *Ancient Egyptian Medicine: The Papyrus Ebers.* Chicago, Ill.: Ares Pub., 1974.

HUGHES, J. Isolation of an endogenous compound from the brain with properties similar to morphine. *Brain Res.* 88: 295–308, 1975.

MOERTEL, C.G. Relief of pain with oral medications. *Aust. N. Z. J. Med.* 6 (Suppl. 1): 1–8, 1976.

MOERTEL, C.G.; AHMANN, D.L.; TAYLOR, W.F.; and SCHWARTAU, N. A comparative evaluation of marketed analgesics. *New England Journal of Medicine* 286: 813–815, 1972.

MOERTEL, C.G.; AHMANN, D.L.; TAYLOR, W.F.; and SCHWARTAU, N. Relief of pain by oral medications. A controlled evaluation of analgesic compounds. *JAMA* 229: 55–59, 1974.

PASTERNAK, G.W.; GOODMAN, R.; and SNYDER, S. H. An endogenous morphine-like factor in mammalian brain. *Life Sciences* 16: 1765–1769, 1975.

YAKSH, T.L.; FARB, D.; LEEMAN, S.; and JESSELL, T. Intrathecal capsaicin depletes substance P in the rat spinal cord and produces prolonged thermal analgesia. *Science* 206: 481–483, 1979.

YAKSH, T.L., and WILSON, P.R. Spinal serotonin terminal system mediates antinociception. *Journal of Pharmacology and Experimental Therapy* 208: 446–453, 1979.

TSOU, K., and JANG, C.S. Studies on the site of analgesic action of morphine by intracerebral microinjection. *Scientia Sinica* 13: 1099–1109, 1964.

11

Surgery for Pain

Herophilus of ancient Egypt knew that some nerves were sensory and others motor (Chapter 2), so it is not surprising that the better informed and more enterprising surgeons of antiquity and the Middle Ages should occasionally have attempted to relieve pain by cutting nerves. Indeed, what could be more reasonable, once it was known that they carried sensation, than to cut them in order to interrupt the painful messages? However, as is so often the case in biology and medicine, what intuitively appears to be logical, in practice may be quite otherwise.

And so it has been with the cutting of nerves, or *neurotomy,* to give it its technical name. Although neurotomies can relieve pain on occasion, it is much more common for failure to result. Furthermore, the number of situations in which neurotomies can be employed is quite limited. Thus, if the pain is restricted to a small area, severing a minor nerve may indeed be adequate. On the other hand, relief of widespread pain would require transection of large nerve trunks, which almost invariably contain important motor components; the resultant paralysis could rarely if ever be justified. Also, loss of all sensation over an extensive area is a more or less unpleasant as well as crippling deficit—especially if the hand is affected, for example. Added to this, it is not unusual for neurotomy to be followed by unpleasant sensations such as pain, burning, and/or tickling, the latter likened by some patients to worms moving under the skin. Since these sensations are spontaneous and more or less constantly present, the discomfort and annoyance may be worse than the pain for which the operation was performed.

Nowadays neurotomies for pain are performed only on rare occasions and after very careful assessment of each situation; temporary block of sensation by injecting a local anesthetic into the affected nerve will give a patient some idea of how well he or she is likely to tolerate the resultant loss of sensation. It also provides some indication of the likelihood of success for a neurotomy; unfortunately, even if the pain is completely relieved in this way on several occasions, there is no guarantee that severing the nerve will give permanent relief. Thus, it is at best an uncertain procedure with quite limited indications.

Dorsal Rhizotomies

In what appears to be the next logical step, surgeons at the end of the nineteenth century began to cut dorsal or sensory roots (see Figure 5.1) for certain types of pain. The rationale seemed excellent, since the sensory fibers are collected in an entirely separate bundle from the motor fibers. It was expected that sensation, including pain, would be abolished while movement would be unimpaired. However, here again results have fallen far short of what logic would predict! Only about a third of patients are permanently relieved of their pain when carefully selected dorsal roots are cut. The other two-thirds have recurrence of their old pain within days to several months.

There are, of course, a number of situations in which severing peripheral nerves or dorsal roots does give immediate and permanent relief of pain, but it is often difficult to predict precisely which patients will be benefited.

OPERATIONS ON THE CENTRAL NERVOUS SYSTEM

As knowledge of the structure and function of the central nervous system was acquired, especially during the last decades of the past century, it gradually became apparent that there were specific pathways for pain; some of that story has been told in Chapter 2. Here the manner in which that information has been applied by surgeons to the treatment of pain is recounted. Until very recently, procedures for the control of pain were purely destructive, and only in the last few years have nondestructive methods been used. The destructive or lesion-producing methods are considered first.

Cordotomy

The operation most commonly performed for the relief of pain due to cancer consists in making a small transverse incision or placing a lesion stereotaxically in the anterior part of the spinal cord. However, because so little was known about the pathways in the central nervous system, and particularly about those conveying noxious signals, it was not until the early years of this century that operations of this type became possible. First it was necessary to know whether there were, in fact, separate pathways for pain and, furthermore, whether such pathways could be severed without producing serious and perhaps lethal complications.

The earliest reliable information about pain tracts in the spinal cord was obtained by Sir William Gowers (1823–1898), one of the great neurologists of the nineteenth century. One day in the summer of 1878, a young Indian student was admitted to his care with a gunshot wound in the neck that had damaged his spinal cord. He survived a little more than a day, but during this time Gowers was much intrigued by the fact that although the patient could move all his limbs without any evidence of weakness and his sense of touch was also intact, he had lost all pain and temperature sensation on one side from the neck down. In addition to being a neurologist, Gowers was also an excellent anatomist, and after the patient died, he carefully examined the spinal cord, finding that the bullet had divided the anterior and lateral aspect of the spinal cord on the side opposite the one that had lost pain and temperature sensation during the patient's brief survival. The conclusion Gowers came to was both simple and logical: Pain and temperature sensations were conducted by a system that ascended in the anterolateral quadrant of the spinal cord on the opposite side; that is, the pathway crossed after entering the cord. Here the matter rested, for this most significant observation passed almost unnoticed.

Then, in 1905, a quarter of a century later, the American neurologist W. G. Spiller (1885–1936) was impressed by the sensory loss he observed in a young tubercular patient: Pain and temperature sensations were almost completely lost on both sides from the neck on down, whereas touch, movement, and reflexes were unaffected. In fact, it was much the same picture as Gowers had described. When Spiller's patient died, two small tubercular masses were found, which had compressed and destroyed the anterior aspect of the spinal cord on each side. Spiller, a forward-looking man, saw the practical implications of his observation and prevailed upon E. Martin (1859–1938), a surgeon, to transect the anterior lateral part of the spinal cord in a patient suffering from severe, unrelenting pain in the pelvis and legs due to cancerous invasion of the lower end of the spinal cord. The operation was performed on the 19th of January, 1911; postoperatively, the patient was markedly relieved of his pain and no longer required morphine. Since that time, many thousands of cordotomies have been done for pains of many types, though mostly for that resulting from cancer.

Unfortunately, cordotomy is not a panacea for pain, for it has certain limitations and complications of which the patient must be fully aware before giving consent for surgery. The main shortcoming of the operation is that the analgesia may not hold up well. Although initial relief is almost invariably complete, at six months, about 30 percent of patients are back to their preoperative situation; at the end of a year, some 50 percent of the patients are again having pain. Of the 50 percent of patients whose pain is still controlled at the end of one year, a small number will have recurrence of pain over the ensuing months. Complete relief of pain for ten or more years is relatively uncommon. Because it is impossible to predict which patients will have prolonged pain relief, the operation is usually advised only for those whose survival is anticipated to be from six months to a year. For patients in this latter group, the relief from unremitting severe pain is an unqualified blessing, allowing them to spend their last days in comparative comfort.

The complications of cordotomy range from rare instances in which a patient succumbs immediately postoperatively to varying degrees of neurological impairment. Insofar as fatality is concerned, any major operation includes this risk. In the case of cordotomy, when both right and left sides were operated on at the same time in the upper part of the cord, a number of patients died because of impairment of the nervous control of breathing; it was subsequently shown that the pathways for this function pass through or near the pain tract. While the patients remained awake, there was no problem, but on falling asleep, some of them "forgot to breathe." Since this problem is now well well recognized, it is rarely if ever an issue, and preventive measures are taken whenever it poses a threat.

Less serious but nevertheless troublesome problems that may occur are a variable degree of weakness in the leg, or arm and leg, on the side of the operation and difficulty with emptying the bladder or controlling the bowels. These disturbances are fortunately of short duration—a few days to a week or so—in most instances. Persistent impairment of genital sensation and, in some cases, weakness of erection also may occur. A small percentage of patients who have undergone this operation may be affected by spontaneous, unpleasant burning, crawling, and even painful sensations in the areas rendered analgesic. Unfortunately, there is little that can be done when this happens.

In summary, as in any irreversible procedure, all these potential complications must be carefully balanced against the very real benefits a cordotomy may provide before a decision is made to proceed.

The operation itself used to require surgical exposure of the spinal cord, following which an incision was made into it with a fine blade. This is rarely done now, having been supplanted by the simpler procedure of inserting an insulated needle, under local anesthesia, through the skin and into the cord under X-ray guidance. Once the uninsulated tip of the needle is precisely positioned in the cord, it is heated by means of a radio-frequency current; as a result, the area of cord surrounding it is coagulated. At this time, to ensure a satisfactory result, the surgeon will carefully check the patient's response to pinprick stimulation; if the lesion is adequate, a pinprick should feel like a touch. Strength in the extremities is also tested repeatedly in order to avoid damage to motor pathways. If the sensory loss is insufficient, the lesion is cautiously enlarged, and the testing procedures are repeated.

Although the procedure as described may seem to be very stressful and unpleasant, most patients tolerate it surprisingly well and are most gratified at the disappearance of their underlying pain.

To conclude, cordotomy is not an ideal solution to the problem of intractable pain, but in carefully selected situations it can provide very significant and even complete relief for periods of six months to a year, and sometimes much longer.

Other Operations for Pain: Stereotaxic Surgery

Since the pain pathway has been traced all the way to the thalamus and the cerebral cortex (Chapter 2), attempts have been made to relieve chronic pain by interrupting it at many levels. Sometimes this was done by exposing it at sites where it could be severed with a scalpel because of its superficial location, and at other times by guiding an electrode into it, using atlases of the brain with precise measurements, complemented with X rays to guide the electrode toward the target zone during the procedure. Such operations are referred to as stereotaxic because guidance in the three spatial planes is required to position the electrode.

For many years the results of these procedures were disappointing; not only did pain return within a short period after initially successful results, but a high incidence of complications, including thalamic pain (see Chapter 8), for which no cure was known, led most surgeons to view them with skepticism.

However, with additional experience accumulated by those surgeons who had the optimism and tenacity to persist in the face of repeated discouragement, much more favorable results are now obtained. Complications are less frequent and pain relief, more predictable and enduring. A recent review of the subject by Sweet (1980) analyzes each of ten different types of operations that have been reported to alleviate pain of advanced cancer. There are several features about these operations that are both surprising and puzzling. For example, whereas chronic, incapacitating pain from cancer is relieved in the successful cases, there is no alteration in such acute pain sensation as being pricked with a pin or exposed to noxious heat. Furthermore, there are at least ten different, widely separated target sites in the brain whose destruction results in relief of pain. A number of these areas have no known connections to the pain pathway, which makes it difficult to understand just how they are involved in the pain experience. It is, of course, theoretically quite possible to get from any point in the central nervous system to any other point, simply because of the incredibly complex nerve network. Thus one could hypothesize that some unknown part of the pain pathway was being interrupted; this is, of course, once again pure speculation and a quite improbable, though possible, explanation.

Another curious feature of these lesions is that pain relief can also be obtained by introducing an electrode into some of the effective sites and then delivering electrical stimulation. In other words, both destruction and stimulation may have the same favorable effect!

Perhaps the most peculiar observation that has been made is that when relief of pain has been obtained by a brain lesion and another pain-producing lesion such as a new metastasis appears subsequently, the new pain is in no way affected by the preexisting brain lesion!

Psychosurgery

The patient suffering from chronic pain has, on one hand, the sensation of pain itself; on the other, he or she has anguish, fear, apprehension, depression, and other distressing emotional symptoms associated with it —globally referred to as the affective component. The proportion between pain sensation and the affective response thereto varies greatly, as discussed in Chapter 1; not infrequently, the affective component becomes of overriding concern, profoundly disrupting the patient's life and turning him or her into an emotional cripple.

These asppect of the pain problem were poorly understood during the first half of this century, and when frontal lobotomy began to be performed in the 1940s and 1950s on patients with chronic pain, many surgeons were persuaded that the operation suppressed pain. The operation itself is technically simple and consists in severing a proportion of the fibers that connect the frontal pole of the brain to the thalamus. Following this operation, patients who had previously required large doses of narcotics for even partial relief no longer complained of pain, nor did they request analgesic drugs; the inference that pain had been suppressed seemed obvious.

At this juncture a personal anecdote relating to my first experience with lobotomy for pain may be quite illuminating. Parenthetically, I claim no particular prescience or clairvoyance with regard to my own reactions, but simply that my observations were made without any preconceptions since, much to my discredit, I had not read the pertinent literature. What I can claim is that my assessment was objective and comparatively accurate. At the time (1950), I was a resident in general surgery in a small hospital. Among the patients under my care was a man of some fifty-five years of age, a chronic smoker, who was suffering from excruciating pain due to metastases from lung cancer that had spread to his left shoulder and involved the large nerve trunks to his arm. He was an intelligent, alert man who had occupied an important executive position. In the brief periods when his pain was at least bearable, he expressed himself in an animated and witty manner; his eyes would sparkle, and a smile would briefly illuminate his face. However, most of the time pain prevented him from engaging in anything but the most essential conversation.

In the hope of easing his existence, I suggested that a neurosurgeon be called to try to relieve his pain with a cordotomy; at the time I was unaware of the fact that cordotomies rarely if ever relieve cancer pain of the upper extremity and especially of the shoulder. For this reason, a bilateral frontal lobotomy, which was much in vogue at the time for the treatment of pain, was done. The operation was carried out without any difficulty, and the patient had an uneventful convalescence. On visiting him the following morning, I was deeply shocked by the change in his appearance: His face was expressionless, and his eyes—which had reflected an active, emotional spirit—were blank, perhaps better described as soulless. When I asked him if he had any pain, to my dismay—for I was responsible for bringing him to this pass—his toneless, monosyllabic answer was "Yes." How could this be? I then inquired whether the pain bothered him. His answer—most surprising to me at the time—was, again in a monotone, "No." Did he want any medicine for his pain? Again the answer was an indifferent "No." He rarely made an effort, either then or during the ensuing weeks of his life, to initiate any conversation or to request anything. His interest in life appeared to have vanished, together with the expression in his face and eyes. The only exception to this was an almost total loss of sexual inhibition, which led him to make both verbal and physical advances toward his nurses; he also urinated in his bed without the least embarrassment. In summary, his general behavior was both slovenly and generally unpleasant. The contrast with his pre-operative personality was frankly appalling.

What can be said for such an operation? First of all, it must be stressed that frontal lobotomies, as practiced at that time, involved very extensive division of the connections between the frontal cortex and major centers in the brain. Furthermore, there was little else to offer patients with chronic, incapacitating pain, though in retrospect, this may seem like a poor justification.

Current Status of Psychosurgery. Because of widespread concern about the negative aspects of psychosurgery, due in part to factual and in part to sensational articles in the press, legislation outlawing such procedures was proposed in the early 1970s. However, Congress took less Draconian measures and instead appointed an eleven-member committee to evaluate and report back on the dangers and benefits, if any, of these operations.

Almost all those who participated in the investigation subsequently recognized that they had approached the task with a more or less pronounced bias against psychosurgery, which was not surprising in view of the serious and often catastrophic side effects of these operations in the early days of psychosurgery, as already described. It was, therefore, most unexpected when the committee returned a very favorable verdict at the end of an exhaustive study. Not only did it recommend that psychosurgery not be banned, but it specifically *encouraged* the Secretary of the Department of Health, Education and Welfare to support research on the subject!

Barbara J. Culliton (1976), of *Science,* the official journal of the American Association for the Advancement of Science, interviewed several members of the committee to ascertain the reasons for the surprising reversal of opinion. Chairman J. Kenneth Ryan of Harvard Medical School was quoted as saying: "We looked at the data and they did not support our prejudices. I, for one, did not expect to come out in favor of psychosurgery. But we saw that some very sick people had been helped by it, and that it did not destroy their intelligence or rob them of their feelings. Their marriages were intact. The operation shouldn't be banned."

Professor Hans-Lukas Teuber, another committee member, stated: "I think I was temperamentally opposed. I was not prepared to see any positive response from patients." But out of eleven patients who had suffered chronic pain with depression, nine were cured, despite having failed to respond previously to the entire gamut of therapy from psychotropic drugs to electroshock. Clearly, such outstanding results could not be disregarded.

Allan F. Mirsky and Maressa H. Orzack carried out a comparable study on twenty-seven patients who had been operated on by one of three neurosurgeons at different centers, each of whom employed differing techniques. As quoted also by Barbara Culliton from a telephone interview with these investigators, who were initially neutral or skeptical about the value of psychosurgery: "When we began seeing the patients, we were just amazed." Fourteen of the twenty-seven patients were considered to have "derived considerable benefit" from psychosurgery, others showed "slight" or "moderate improvement," and none suffered any deleterious side effects.

Psychosurgery is rarely advised nowadays, since remarkable improvements in drug therapy for anxiety and depression provide equally satisfactory and often better results without the risk of irreversible deficits, though some toxic effects do occur. Furthermore, improved management of chronic pain by drugs, stimulation, and other procedures has relegated psychosurgery for pain to a secondary position. However—and this is the crucial point, well brought out in the conclusions of the congressional panel—there are some situations in which patients with chronic, incapacitating pain cannot be benefited by any of the commonly available pharmacological or operative procedures. It is for these people and for a limited number of patients with obsessive-compulsive neuroses or depression with or without pain, those who are completely refractory to any of the psychotropic drugs, that psychosurgery may provide relief not available in any other way.

These procedures should, however, be performed only in a few highly specialized centers because of the need for very careful screening of patients who may be candidates for surgery, and because the results should be studied in particular depth and detail in order to obtain the maximum information possible about brain function both during and after the operation and thus to provide an invaluable data bank for the future.

Cingulumotomy

A more recently developed operation, cingulumotomy consists in severing a bundle of fibers—the cingulum—that follows a ringlike course around the center of the brain, connecting the frontal cortex with the limbic cortex. Because of these connections between areas of the brain concerned with emotions, it was felt that cutting it might help to alleviate the anxiety and fear associated with chronic pain. Opinions remain divided regarding its effectiveness; it is a relatively simple procedure with minor operative risks and carries with it no detectable impairment of personality. As in the case of frontal lobotomy, it is most effective in cases of intractable obsessive-compulsive neurosis and depression.

Hypophysectomy

Some twenty-five years ago, the Swedish neurosurgeons Luft and Olivecrona removed the pituitary gland (hypophysis) from a number of patients suffering from advanced, inoperable cancer of the breast in the hope of altering the hormonal balance and thus retarding or even curing the tumor. Progression of the tumor was markedly slowed in a number of instances, but perhaps the most remarkable observation was that pain was often strikingly reduced or actually suppressed!

Since that time much experience has been acquired with hypophysectomy for pain due to inoperable tumors arising from glands (breast, ovary, prostate) that are regulated to some extent by pituitary hormones and from others that are non-hormone-dependent. The results have been, in general, favorable, with rapid and, at times, immediate postoperative disappearance of pain. The relief of pain has frequently lasted for many months and up to a year or more in some instances. The reason for this is still obscure, though several hypotheses have been proposed. Sweet has emphasized that when hypophysectomy has been done by injection of alcohol into the gland, damage to adjacent parts of the hypothalamus may account for the relief of pain.

Others have suggested that there may be some change in endorphin levels as a result of the pituitary destruction. This suggestion is based on the fact that beta lipoprotein, which is formed by the pituitary, contains the amino acid sequence of enkephalin, which (as discussed in Chapter 10) has been shown to have powerful analgesic properties comparable to those of morphine. Why destruction of the pituitary with consequent loss of endorphin production should relieve or suppress pain is, however, not readily explained. We have here another instance in which new and important knowledge has been acquired that has, in turn, raised a series of other questions for which we as yet have no answers.

FUNCTIONAL (PHYSIOLOGICAL) OPERATIONS FOR PAIN: STIMULUS-PRODUCED ANALGESIA

Until very recently, operations for the relief of pain were limited to interrupting pathways or making lesions in nuclei of the nociceptive and related systems. The optimal lesion had to be accurately placed and no larger than absolutely necessary to obtain the desired result. Even in expert hands, these requirements are often difficult to meet due to the normal variations in measurements of the brain. An issue of particular importance is the irreversibility of such lesions in the brain. Whereas other organs have pronounced regenerative powers, nerve cells have lost this ability; and though nerve fibers in the brain are capable of some regeneration, this is inadequate—both in extent and quality—to reestablish lost function. Thus, there is no recovery, and no return to the preoperative situation is possible in the event of an error. Furthermore, the minor degree of regeneration that does occur may be actually disadvantageous, since it may be the cause of the unpleasant and sometimes painful sensations termed *dysesthesiae.*

For these and other reasons, the emphasis has shifted in recent years to more physiological operations aimed at stimulating pathways that are known to depress or inhibit pain, such as the descending inhibitory systems described in Chapter 2. Although the existence of such systems had been suspected for many years, experimental proof first appeared in the 1950s. Since then, a great deal of information has been acquired; some of it has been applied with success to some types of human pain that previously had been refractory to all available treatment. Various names have been used to describe this new type of surgery, including stimulus-produced analgesia (SPA) and neuroaugmentative surgery.

Experience with this type of treatment is quite recent, and in the more complex and intractable pain problems, a number of years must elapse before conclusions regarding therapeutic validity can be arrived at. Thus, the long-term effectiveness of these procedures is still somewhat uncertain. A point of major importance in appraising these methods is that they are used to treat the most difficult and intractable pain problems; patients who have had extensive trials with every type of analgesic and/or psychotropic drug and, not infrequently, one or more of the standard operations for pain without obtaining any relief are the formidable challenge the new operations have to face. This includes patients with chronic, incapacitating low back pain who have been unable to obtain relief after multiple operations, patients with pain from amputations of limbs, and others with pain due to hemorrhages or other lesions in the central nervous system.

The basis of the operation is to stimulate either the periaqueductal gray area, the sensory nucleus of the thalamus, or the internal capsule (a massive bundle of nerve fibers in the center of the brain that contains sensory and motor fibers; see Chapter 2), which—as shown by past experience—are effective targets for inducing pain relief. Electrical stimulation requires insertion of a long, metal needle (steel, tungsten, silver, or other metal is used), which is insulated except for its tip, to reach targets deep in the brain, as previously described for stereotaxic brain lesions.

A question often asked is whether there is not great danger of serious and disabling damage to the brain from piercing it this way—to its very depths. The fact is that the amount of damage caused by a needle approximately 1 mm in diameter is, with very rare exceptions, quite negligible. This is because, on one hand, a location is selected in the cerebral cortex for the needle's point of entrance where no detectable deficit results from such a puncture. On the other hand, and surprisingly enough, although many fibers and neurons are damaged, the relative proportion is so small that no adverse effects occur. An ever-present, though fortunately rare, complication is that a blood vessel, especially a small artery, may be punctured, in which case the resultant hemorrhage can have serious consequences. Again, operations of this type are only carried out as a last resort in patients who are desperate for any form of relief, some of whom even threaten suicide unless something is done for them. Thus, certain grave, though calculated, risks have to be taken in such serious and gloomy situations.

Once the electrode has been successfully positioned, it is connected to an electronic stimulator positioned underneath the skin in an area that can easily be reached by the patient, who is shown how to use an external device that he or she places over the buried stimulator to activate it. Stimulation is done for periods of up to twenty minutes at a time, and the current and frequency are adjustable for obtaining the optimal effect. Interestingly, pain is relieved in some patients for a number of hours and even days following the end of stimulation.

The results of SPA of the brain have been spectacularly successful in some cases of pain that was resistant to all other treatment. The pain has disappeared or decreased so markedly as to be quite tolerable; and, particularly important, the procedure has continued to be effective for many months, and up to five years in some reports.

Several problems have been encountered, among them failure of the stimulator, an event that is rapidly detected by the patient and easily remedied. More worrisome is the fact that tolerance to stimulation tends to occur; this is similar to tolerance to morphine and other drugs in that over a period of time, the same intensity of stimulation becomes progressively less effective, requiring higher currents to achieve the same degree of pain relief. This problem can be diminished to some extent by keeping the frequency of stimulation periods to a minimum compatible with comfort and, sometimes, by discontinuing stimulation for a day or two, after which tolerance appears to have diminished. However, it can be expected to build up again on return to regular use of the stimulator. It is ironic that with each new advance in the therapy of pain, some new problem almost invariably appears, as exemplified by the development of tolerance in this instance and by the similar problem with the enkephalins, as described in Chapter 10.

Electrical Stimulation of Nerves

There are many situations in which pain is restricted to a peripheral nerve, and it would be quite unreasonable to treat it by a complex and potentially hazardous technique such as that just described. For patients in this situation, the more simple methods of stimulating peripheral nerves have proven to be useful in selected instances.

Peripheral nerve stimulation therapy stemmed conceptually from the gate control theory of Melzack and Wall (see Chapter 2). Since one of the principal postulates of the theory was that activity in large-diameter sensory fibers blocked or gated the central effects of fine fibers (which carry noxious signals), Wall and Sweet (1967) reasoned that it should be possible to control pain by taking advantage of this antagonism. By one of those rare and fortunate circumstances, it just so happens that large-diameter nerve fibers have a much lower threshold to electrical stimulation than do fine fibers, and thus it is possible to activate them selectively. When a pulsed stimulating current was delivered to the sensory nerves, a sensation of vibration was felt as the current was applied, and when the right stimulus frequency and intensity were delivered to the nerve of a volunteer, pain sensation was depressed. More important was the finding that when this type of stimulation was applied to the appropriate nerve of patients with chronic pain, striking relief was obtained in a significant proportion of cases.

The surgical procedure is relatively straightforward and consists in placing a cuff containing the electrodes around the nerve that has been selected on the basis of clinical examination and diagnostic tests. The conducting leads from the electrodes are led beneath the tissues to a point where the stimulating device or receiver is implanted. The location of the latter will depend on the nerve to be stimulated (i.e., upper or lower extremity) and is planned to provide as much comfort and accessibility as possible. The receiver is activated by a small transmitter that operates on radio-frequency current. The patient places the antenna of the transmitter directly over the buried receiver and then adjusts the current and frequency to obtain the optimum result.

With careful selection, approximately 50 percent of patients with a variety of otherwise intractable painful conditions have obtained relief of their pain for periods of years; it is, of course, necessary to stimulate the nerve at frequent intervals each day. Interestingly, stimulation of the nerve for periods of fifteen to twenty minutes at a time often provides relief for several hours and sometimes for considerably longer periods. Tingling or vibrating sensations are noted when the stimulator is activated, but most patients find these sensations entirely tolerable.

It is also possible to stimulate peripheral nerves through the skin by placing electrodes over points where a nerve comes near the surface. This technique is called transcutaneous electrical nerve stimulation (TENS) and, other than the operative procedure, has advantages and disadvantages similar to those of direct nerve stimulation.

Dorsal Column Stimulation

Based also on the gate control theory, this method of treating pain was introduced in 1970 by Shealy and associates. The dorsal columns are the massive bundles of fibers that form the dorsal or posterior part of the spinal cord (see Figure 3.8). Since these tracts are composed of large-caliber myelinated fibers, Shealy employed the same rationale as Sweet and Wall; that is, he hypothesized that if the large fibers were stimulated, their discharges would block the input from small "pain"-signaling fibers.

The results of this technique have been less satisfactory than those of TENS, and opinions remain divided about its value in treating chronic, intractable pain problems. At this time it is perhaps best to regard it as an experimental technique whose virtues are yet to be established.

REFERENCES

CULLITON, B.J. Psychosurgery: National commission issues surprisingly favorable report. *Science* 194: 299–301, 15 October 1976. Copyright 1976 by the American Association for the Advancement of Science.

GOWERS, W. A case of unilateral gunshot injury to the spinal cord. *Tran. Clin. Soc. London* 11: 24–32, 1878.

LOESER, J.D., BLACK, R. G., and CHRISTMAN, R. N. Relief of pain by transcutaneous stimulation. *Journal of Neurosurgery* 42: 308–314, 1975.

LONG, D.L., and ERICKSON, D.E. Stimulation of the posterior columns of the spinal cord for the relief of intractable pain. *Surgical. Neurology* 4: 134–141, 1975.

LONG, D.M., and HAGFORS, N. Electrical stimulation of the nervous system: The current status. *Pain* 1: 109–123, 1975.

NASHOLD, B.S., and FRIEDMAN, H. Dorsal column stimulation for the control of pain. Preliminary report on 30 patients. *Journal of Neurosurgery* 36: 590–597, 1972.

SHEALY, C.N.: MORTIMER, J.T., and HAGFORS, N.R. Dorsal column electroanalgesia. *Journal of Neurosurgery* 32: 560–564, 1970.

SPILLER, W.G., and MARTIN, E. The treatment of persistent pain of organic origin in the lower part of the body by division of the anterolateral column of the spinal cord. *JAMA* 58: 1489–1490, 1912.

SWEET, W.H. Central mechanisms of chronic pain (neuralgias and certain other neurogenic pain). In Pain, *Res. Pub. Ass. Res. Nerv. Ment. Dis.* 58: 287–303, 1980.

WALL, P.D., and SWEET, W.H. Temporary abolition of pain in man. *Science* 155: 108–109, 1967.

WHITE, J.C., and SWEET, W.H. *Pain and the neurosurgeon.* Springfield, Ill.: Charles C. Thomas, 1969, 1000 pp.

12

Acupuncture and Pain

Acupuncture originated in China several thousand years ago, where it was used to treat a wide variety of disorders—from colic to arthritis, epilepsy to headaches. Because some of these complaints have a fluctuating or intermittent course, it has always been difficult to determine whether relief was due to the treatment or to a natural remission of the disorder. Physicians have usually taken the latter point of view and looked upon it as one of the less dangerous forms of quackery.

It appears to have been introduced to the Western world by Ten Rhyne, a Dutch physician of the seventeenth century; since then, it has enjoyed periods of popularity such as the one that occurred in France and Germany during the 1930s. However, over a hundred years ago, as astute a clinical observer as Silas Weir Mitchell, commenting on his experiences with the wounded from the Civil War, stated: "Of acupuncture in traumatic neuralgia, I have nothing good to say; it was repeatedly used by our staff, without the slightest advantage. . . ." More recently, resurgence of interest began with a report by James Reston, a correspondent of the *New York Times*, who was operated on for appendicitis while in China covering President Nixon's trip in 1972. He received acupuncture treatment for postoperative abdominal pain and wrote an eloquent testimonial on the very significant relief he experienced. It is important to note that acupuncture *was not used* for analgesic purposes during the operation itself.

Regardless of the details, an enthusiastic endorsement from an experienced international correspondent inevitably evoked widespread excitement. Although some were skeptical, many concluded that an innocuous and efficient method of combating pain might be at hand. In view of this and numerous subsequent reports—some of them quite startling—attesting to the usefulness of the method, it is of more than passing interest to take a close look at this strange phenomenon and to try to weigh the conflicting evidence as dispassionately as possible.

WHAT IS ACUPUNCTURE?

The traditional method of administering acupuncture consists in introducing one or more slender bamboo needles through the skin and into the underlying muscle at carefully selected sites. Once the needle point is considered to be accurately positioned, the acupuncturist begins to twirl it rapidly back and forth with a rotary motion between thumb and fingers; in the case of surgical procedures, this may go on for several hours.

The selection of the site at which needles are to be inserted is regarded as extremely important by acupuncturists and is governed to a great extent by charts, some of which date back several centuries. These charts show a series of lines called "meridians" on which small circles are inscribed at intervals. The latter represent the acupuncture "points." Whether the meridians and points have any value is doubtful at best.

Acupuncturists, however, adhere quite strictly to this ancient methodology and use specific points to treat particular disorders; in the case of patients with pain, the "point" bears a special relationship to the site of the discomfort. For example, pain in the head or face is almost always treated by activating the Hoku point—that is, a point near the base of the thumb on the dorsal aspect of the hand. Interestingly, if one has a unilateral headache, considerable or even complete transient relief can often be obtained by pressing this area firmly until a moderately painful sensation is felt.

When a satisfactory result is obtained, the subject remains fully conscious, and is able to converse and execute movements without any apparent limitation but, strikingly, appears to be quite indifferent to stimuli that, under normal circumstances, would be excruciatingly painful. This is especially noteworthy in surgical procedures carried out with no other method of pain control than acupuncture, as described later in this chapter.

The traditional manually rotated bamboo needles are often replaced nowadays by electrical acupuncture. This consists in introducing steel needles at the same sites and delivering pulsed electrical stimulation. The results obtained are similar, and the convenience—especially in operations that last for one to two hours—is obvious.

ACUPUNCTURE IN SURGERY

Reports that surgical operations were being carried out on human patients in China with acupuncture as the sole method of pain control were received by most Western physicians with the greatest skepticism. I admit to being among the incredulous, being quite certain that those who claimed to have witnessed such remarkable events must have been either extremely naïve or carried away by that curious willingness to accept the most improbable assertions as factual that seems to seize some visitors to exotic new environments. The People's Republic of China (PRC) was most certainly mysterious and exotic, not only because China has always had such an aura but also because it had been off limits to most foreigners for thirty years.

It was, therefore, with a mixture of excitement and profound curiosity that I visited the PRC in 1974 as a member of a scientific study group to try to assess the value of acupuncture as an *anesthetic* in surgery. I emphasize the term *anesthetic* to point out that it is incorrectly, though commonly, applied; under no circumstances has acupuncture produced anesthesia—that is, loss of sensation. Patients receiving acupuncture preserve touch and probably most other sensations. What appears to be modified in favorable instances is some aspect of pain sensation. Therefore the effect should be referred to as acupuncture *analgesia*.

The data gathered during that fascinating visit have been summarized and published by the National Academy of Sciences of the United States, which underwrote and sponsored the project in conjunction with the Chinese Medical Association. Both organizations provided every assistance to the visiting team; some details of the manner in which information was obtained and evaluated are herewith summarized in order that the reader may draw his or her own conclusions as to the reliability of observations.

For every operation, a three-page checklist was filled out either during or immediately after the procedure by three (or more) members of the group. The lists were exhaustive and included everything from the patient's age, sex, and occupation to the preoperative and postoperative diagnosis; whether pain medication, tranquilizers, or other drugs had been given before or during the procedure; and whether there was any evidence of suffering during the operation. Each observation was thoroughly discussed and the corresponding statement agreed upon by the three or more observers present at the operation. Finally, an overall grade was given that was unanimously agreed upon and the protocol signed by all observers of the operation.

The grading system was as follows:

Grade I	(a) No signs of discomfort at any time. (b) Only standard premedication or small amount of opiate given prior to operation. (c) No local anesthetic administered during the operation.
Grade II	(a) Mild and transient signs of discomfort, but procedure clearly tolerable by an average individual. (b) Small amount of analgesic drugs given, but entirely insufficient by themselves to provide surgical analgesia.
Grades III & IV	(a) Obvious evidence of pain. (b) Need for local or general anesthetic to be able to complete procedure. (c) Morphine, Demerol, tranquilizers also given in considerable quantities. (d) Clearly an "analgesic" failure.

When the results were analyzed and tabulated on return to the United States, all the information required was available; in other words, the questionnaires had been entirely adequate for the purpose and had been completed in every instance. Before considering the conclusions reached by the study group as a whole, some comments on the attitude toward acupuncture of the one member for whom I can speak—myself—may be of some value to the reader.

Briefly, I had paid little or no attention to it until the report by Reston. At that point I concluded that the benefits, if any, were almost certainly of a psychological nature and probably enhanced by the unusual environment; perhaps even, shall we say, a worldly and case-hardened reporter suffering considerable discomfort might be less than entirely objective in his judgement under the special circumstances at the time.

However, as I note later in paragraphs on the scientific basis for acupuncture, my skepticism was rather rudely shaken shortly before traveling to the PRC by an experiment carried out to demonstrate that acupuncture was nothing more than quackery or a placebo effect.

Despite being somewhat chastened by this experience, I was still very dubious that acupuncture was of any value in situations in which severe pain would be anticipated and particularly so in the case of major surgical operations. Although I cannot be as categorical about the attitude of the other members of the study group, I believe it is fair to say that in general, they were similarly skeptical. A common point of view, however, was that the assessment would be as objective and unprejudiced as possible, with every effort made to determine whether patients were "brainwashed" into some kind of quasi-religious fervor during which they might be oblivious to pain; the stories of patients being wheeled into operating rooms with rapt expressions on their faces as they joyously waved Chairman Mao's little red book were quite prevalent at the time. Or perhaps they were under the effects of hypnotic suggestion, or possibly they were specially selected for their stoicism; there were, indeed, numerous possibilities to be considered.

What we did see and how we attempted to interpret our observations were far removed from what we had anticipated and are perhaps best conveyed by describing some of the experiences. The first operation carried out with acupuncture analgesia alone, which we observed, was performed at the Peking Tuberculosis Research Hospital. We arrived at 8:00 A.M., and after the customary introductions and formalities, we were shown the chest X rays of the patient who was to be operated on. These showed a very clear-cut cavitary lesion in the upper lobe of the right lung. We were then issued gowns, clean linen boots, caps, and masks and were conducted to the operating room, which was quite similar to those in most city hospitals in the United States.

Standing beside the operating table, dressed in the standard Mao jacket, pants, and slippers, was the patient, a slight man of forty years who was obviously quite at ease as he shook hands with the visitors and smilingly answered our carefully rehearsed "Ni hao" (How are you?) with the customary "Hen hao" (Very well). The patient then stripped off his jacket, climbed up on the table, and lay on his left side in the position requested, exposing his right chest—front, side, and back. While the skin was being washed with antiseptic soap and drapes applied, the acupuncturist had inserted thin steel acupuncture needles into both ankles and wrists and had begun stimulation with electrical pulses. After twenty minutes of this, he looked up at the surgeon and nodded, whereupon—and without more ado—the latter took a scalpel and made a twelve-inch-long incision through the patient's skin, following almost the entire length of the interspace between two ribs. In accordance with prior agreements, each of the visiting observers had specific assignments, taking motion pictures or stills, observing, and making notes of the patient's facial expression and, when possible, changes in the pupillary diameter—dilatation being a good and involuntary indication of pain—recording blood pressure, respiratory rate, and so on. Since only one patient was being operated on at this time, there were more than sufficient observers, and considerable overlap in documentation occurred.

Had the patient sat up with a loud scream as the knife blade sliced through his skin, no one would have been particularly surprised. But, astonishingly, he showed not the slightest sign that anything unusual had occurred, continuing to look around, smile, and answer questions in the most relaxed manner. I happened to be watching his face from a distance of some two feet and detected no twitch, no quiver or change in expression. If there were any changes in expression, they were exhibited by the visitors, though one could hardly tell in view of the surgical masks. It is no exaggeration to say that one and all were profoundly moved by this first personal experience with acupuncture analgesia. The initial moments of almost stunned surprise quickly gave way to great excitement as the pent-up curiosity of several months of speculation was finally being satisfied. It should be said, to the great credit of the surgeon who was performing the operation, that he proceeded quite unflustered by the incessant flashes, clicks, and whirring of cameras.

The operation continued smoothly, bleeding vessels in the skin and muscle being coagulated with the electrocautery; the thoracic cavity was opened and the ribs spread widely to allow easy access to the lung, still without the least sign of pain. Equally astonishing to the visitors was the fact that despite the collapse of the right lung, the patient was able to breathe without assistance using the left lung. Parenthetically, it is noted that thoracic surgery had been delayed for many years because of the problems associated with pneumothorax—this is, entrance of air at atmospheric pressure into the chest cavity. It was believed that this would result in death from the collapse of both lungs. Although more or less complex methods were developed toward the end of the nineteenth century to allow surgical access to the lung, the development of positive-pressure gas anesthesia using a well-fitting, cuffed endotracheal tube had finally resolved the problem in the 1920s. Clearly, the patient we were observing was able to breathe only in a marginal fashion, but it was, nevertheless, sufficient for the operation to be completed!

Meanwhile, the surgeon had identified the major vessels and bronchus (pedicle) supplying the upper lobe of the lung, which, as noted, contained the tuberculous cavity. At this point a clamp was applied to the pedicle; this resulted in an access of coughing that quickly subsided. The lobe was then removed, the pedicle tied off, and the chest cavity closed with a tube left in place to aspirate air and secretions. Once the skin incision had been sutured and a dressing applied, the patient sat up by himself and, smiling broadly, proceeded to put on and button up his pajama jacket without assistance. Figure 12.1(*a*) shows the patient at this time; moments later he shook hands with me with a firm grasp and was wheeled out of the operating room. There was no argument about giving him a grade of I on our scale!

Figure 12.1. Major operations done with acupuncture analgesia in the People's Republic of China in 1974.

(a) This man had just had a thoractomy with removal of the right upper lobe of his lung.

(b) A smiling patient whose stomach was being removed at this moment. Acupuncture was administered with bamboo needles.

(c) Splitting of the sternum and removal of an orange-sized tumor (thymoma) from the chest made this patient look a little tired.

(d) A congenital malformation of the heart (interventricular septal defect) was repaired in this young teacher; tubes from the extracorporeal pump–oxygenator can be seen running into the heart in the lower part of the photograph.

Photograph (*d*) by kind permission of Dr. Jerome Modell.

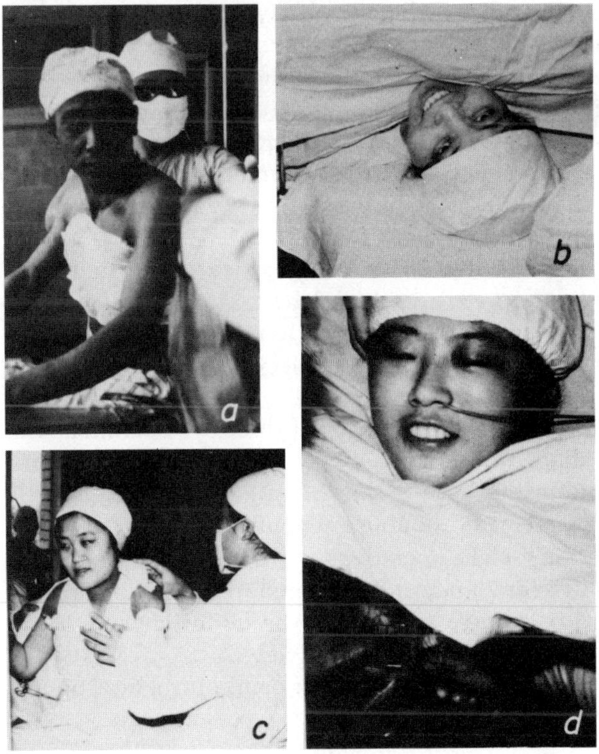

Points of particular relevance are that this patient received no premedication (either opiate analgesics such as morphine or sedatives) and that no local anesthetic was administered during the operation. Futhermore, he was fully alert at all times and showed no trace of the vacant, staring gaze characteristic of the patient under hypnosis. Obviously, someone might object that premedication had indeed been administered prior to the arrival of the observers. However, there is no known analgesic drug that will totally control all signs of pain—as was the case in this and other operations we witnessed—without producing more or less profound clouding of consciousness and confusion, neither of which were observed. Neither at this time nor at any subsequent moment did we have any reason to believe that anything was being hidden from us; we received frank and detailed answers to our questions and were permitted great liberty in observing all aspects of the proceedings.

Other equally striking successes of acupuncture analgesia were observed during the three-week visit. For example, a twenty-two-year-old woman [Figure 12.1(*d*)] had her ventriculoseptal defect (a hole between the left and right main cavities of the heart) operated on with no observable sign of discomfort and was also given a grade of I. The procedure entails splitting the sternum (breastbone) longitudinally using an electrically powered reciprocating saw and placing the patient on extracorporeal circulation—that is, a heart pump, oxygenator, and heat exchanger. She received as premedication 50 mg of Demerol and 100 mg of barbiturate, a combination of drugs that would be totally inadequate to control the pain of suturing a small cut let alone that of major surgery. This patient was fully conscious throughout the procedure and smiled, apparently effortlessly, as she was taken to the recovery room.

Among other major operations that were carried out without evidence of significant discomfort were a subtotal gastrectomy, graded I [Figure 12.1 (*b*)]; a thoracotomy with removal of a thymoma, graded I [Figure 12.1 (*c*)]; two appendectomies, graded II; a cholecystectomy, graded II; a hysterectomy, graded I; an ovariectomy, graded I; and five thyroidectomies for benign tymors, grades I, I, I, II, and II. Each of three eye operations was graded I, and three orthopedic operations—an arthrodesis (grade II) and two ruptured ligaments in the knee (grade I each)—were done entirely successfully with minor premedication and acupuncture alone.

Out of a total of forty-eight operations witnessed, the study group concluded that thirty-five (or 73 percent) appeared to have had either no pain at all (45 percent) or pain so minor as to be quite tolerable to the average individual in our own society. There were thirteen cases (or 27 percent) that were regarded as failures in terms of pain control by acupuncture; in these instances liberal administration of local anesthetics and of analgesic drugs was required in order to complete the operation.

From the preceding description, it must be apparent that something quite remarkable was indeed occurring: A group of experienced observers, each of whom had expertise in one or more aspects of the pain problem, was allowed free access to the patients during the whole of the operative procedure and concluded that in approximately 75 percent of all instances, pain appeared to be either absent or minimal under conditions where it would be expected to be agonizing and unbearable!

However, despite the most lengthy and searching discussions, held both as a part of the study group's duties and during impromptu conversations, it was quite impossible to account for these remarkable observations by recourse to what is known about pain mechanisms. Neither neurophysiologic, psychologic, nor any other scientific argument shed any light on these carefully observed phenomena. As noted earlier, there was no evidence whatsoever of hypnosis being responsible; nor, insofar as could be determined, was there any state of emotional exaltation such as has been said to account for the apparent imperviousness to pain of religious and other martyrs burned at the stake and otherwise tormented. In summary, our study group could find no logical explanation for what we saw. However, the fact that a scientific explanation could not be given is, of itself, no basis for rejecting an analgesic action in acupuncture, since (as discussed in Chapter 9) the mechanism by which general anesthetics exert their effects is still unresolved.

Of much more immediate and pragmatic interest, however, is the question of the potential usefulness of acupuncture analgesia in surgery, either as a substitute or adjunct to currently used anesthetics. Since the latter are all toxic to a variable extent and because, moreover, some patients tolerate anesthetics poorly, acupuncture would appear to offer an ideal method of relieving pain without the risk of untoward drug reactions. This theoretically appealing reasoning runs into several major problems. The first is that only a small percentage of the population can be rendered pain free or, at least, sufficiently analgesic to allow a surgical procedure to be performed. Even in China, where the method has been used in several hundred thousand operations, only a little over 10 percent of patients are found to be suitable candidates for acupuncture analgesia. The determination of suitability hinges, to a major degree, on preoperative screening by the acupuncturist, who must be able to elicit a phenomenon termed *teh-chi.* This is evoked in susceptible candidates by inserting and twirling or electrically activating a needle in a selected acupuncture point; the satisfactory response consists in a feeling of soreness, swelling, heaviness, and numbness in the needled area while the acupuncturist detects a sensation "as if the needle had been grasped by the muscle." Further attrition in the number of successful cases occurs when the method is put to the test, for, as noted, failures occur during surgery in some 25 percent of the carefully screened candidates.

From a purely practical point of view, furthermore, there is a period of some twenty minutes during which the acupuncturist induces analgesia, and there is, as stated, no guarantee that the desired result will be obtained; whereas with general anesthesia, the result is not in doubt. To this must be added the major disruption and potential hazards that may be incurred if, in mid-operation, it becomes necessary to switch to general anesthesia because pain is not being suppressed by acupuncture.

A further limitation of acupuncture for surgery is that it is only marginally successful in some areas of the body. For example, though excellent results were observed in operations on the thyroid and often in chest operations, abdominal operations had to be carried out with extreme gentleness, and failure to control pain was quite frequent, though even here some remarkable successes were seen.

At this time all the evidence indicates that acupuncture analgesia for surgery is an interesting or, even better, a striking and poorly understood phenomenon, which may or may not have potential usefulness in the future. However, it can only be considered as experimental, and indeed it is so regarded in China. For it to gain general acceptance in the operating room, it will have to be developed much further, to the point where a much larger percentage of the population can be rendered pain free. Whether it is possible to train individuals to respond better or in some other way to improve the predictability of a satisfactory result is entirely a matter of speculation. Hypnosis, which has several of the same limitations as acupuncture for analgesia, has not advanced appreciably in methodology or acceptance, though it has been employed quite extensively for some two centuries. However, significant advances in understanding the mechanisms of hypnosis have been made in recent years (Chapter 13).

One issue that surfaces quite frequently is the possibility that differences in racial or societal attitudes toward pain may account for the apparent effectiveness of acupuncture analgesia as observed by Westerners in China. Although this may be a factor of some significance, it seems unlikely that it plays a major role, since similar effects have been reported on a number of occasions by Caucasian volunteers in the Western world. A rather striking example of this was published by a Scandinavian study group that visited China in 1973; one of the delegation, Dr. Birger Nygaard-Ostby, Professor of Dentistry at the University of Oslo, gave the following description of his own experience with acupuncture:

When I returned to Norway, I decided to try acupuncture analgesia myself when my second upper molar had to be removed. Dr. Eric Hoel carried out the acupuncture, inserting the needles at the ho-ku point (Li4) in both hands, and connecting them with a battery stimulator. At first, I felt a little twitching in the muscles of the hand, and then the te-chi feeling. After 10 minutes the dentist loosened the gingiva, which is very sensitive, around the tooth, and I felt no pain. The luxation and extraction were carried out very slowly according to my own wish, and during the entire operation there was no pain whatsoever, even if I, in an inexplicable way, could feel the periodontal fibers being severed.

ACUPUNCTURE AS MEDICAL TREATMENT

The long tradition of treating a large variety of disorders by acupuncture in China and Japan naturally led to its use in the Western world. In recent years the great proliferation of practitioners and clinics employing this mode of treatment raises some important questions about its validity. Can a well-balanced and essentially fair judgment be reached, based on available information? Or should it simply be shrugged off as just another fad and lumped together with folk remedies, iridology, faith healing, and similar pseudosciences?

Acupuncture for Chronic Pain?

The easiest and safest answer would be to reject it formally and to emphasize the anecdotal nature of most of the claims made for it and its lack of scientific underpinnings. However, this in itself would be a chauvinistic and nonscientific approach. In the case of general anesthesia, for example, which no one would question, there is still no adequate scientific explanation for the phenomenon; yet it has been in use for over a century in what we proudly regard as a scientifically based medical system! Furthermore, there is some experimental evidence that acupuncture can indeed produce significant functional alterations in the central nervous system (see pages 167 and those following).

And, of course, there are many reports of remarkable alleviation of chronic pain by acupuncture when all else has failed. An example of this is the following case, treated by my colleague Dr. Josef Wang, who generously furnished the details that follow:

CASE REPORT (0-748-312)

A 57-year-old white female underwent radical mastectomy in 1970 because of adenocarcinoma of the left breast. Shortly after the surgery, she began to suffer from chest wall pain which radiated into the left upper extremity. Cobalt 60 treatment was instituted and on several occasions left T3, T4 and T5 somatic nerve blocks were carried out without relief of pain. She was then placed on both non-narcotic and narcotic analgesics and obtained partial pain relief.

She was seen at the Pain Clinic in 1973 with persistent pain involving the left chest wall, axillary region, and the upper arm. A thorough evaluation at that time revealed no recurrence of the malignacy. A series of acupuncture treatments were performed by applying electrical stimulation (a symmetrical waveform, 5 to 10 Hertz, maximal tolerable current) at sites over the distribution of the left brachial plexus and peripheral nerves of the upper extremity. She obtained complete pain relief which lasted for a few weeks. Although pain recurred, she continued to obtain substantial relief from subsequent acupuncture treatments.

In 1978, she experienced progressive increase in pain in the left chest wall and upper arm. A left pleural effusion was detected. There was a metastatic lesion to the brachial plexus and left chest wall. She was placed on a mixture of narcotics, tranquilizers, and sedatives. She expired in May of 1979.

Comment: During a period of five years, acupuncture therapy was most effective in relieving her pain. Although pain recurred, she responded well to acupuncture treatments on repeated occasions. Attention is drawn to the fact that pain relief persisted for several weeks after the end of the acupuncture series.

Though such successes are not frequent, there is no doubt that they do indeed occur, some having been observed and reported by individuals whose reliability cannot be questioned. Why should acupuncture be successful when other methods, which have received the seal of approval of conventional medical practice, have failed? We do not know, but it is also only fair to remember that a much larger proportion of patients with pain who fail to respond to acupuncture therapy do respond to conventional medical treatment. However, since that is less surprising, they receive far less attention.

Acupuncture in Chronic Pain: Treatment or Illusion? The anguish and, indeed, the desperation of the patient with chronic pain who has spent much money and time in a fruitless search for relief by conventional methods can only be understood by others in a like situation or by a truly sympathectic relative, friend, or physician. Should a patient in this situation turn to acupuncture, and if so, what are the prospects for relief?

The first and obvious answer is that since, for one reason or another, usually accepted methods of treatment are of no avail, why not try acupuncture? It is difficult to muster any good arguments for or against this viewpoint; little or, more probably, no harm is likely to result from the treatment, the only negative aspect being the financial one in the event of another failure. The real question is, What is the likelihood of obtaining significant and enduring relief? Unfortunately, this question cannot be answered, since no well-controlled study of the success or failure rate of acupuncture for chronic pain has been published. Other factors are the difficulty of carrying out such a study in a manner whereby observer bias is minimal or absent, the problem of comparing cases of chronic pain whose individual characteristics are so varied, and, finally, the role of placebo effects. The acupuncturists themselves find it very difficult to respond to these issues and criticisms.

In summary, at this time there are insufficient data to support claims that acupuncture can provide relief for chronic pain other than what can be attributed to the placebo effect. However, striking successes such as the one reproduced in this chapter and numerous anecdotal reports of prolonged relief of pain indicated that the procedure should not be written off.

A SCIENTIFIC BASIS FOR ACUPUNCTURE?

By and large, for a drug or new treatment to acquire acceptance and respectability, it should meet certain logical standards. Obviously, it must be shown to confer certain benefits on the individual being treated, and optimally, experiments should show how it works and, if possible, provide a quantitative measure of the effects claimed for it.

In the case of acupuncture, as already noted, it is very difficult to obtain evidence that would convince a majority of observers that it does, in fact, relieve pain. There is no point in trying to convince everyone, since even the most rigid "proofs" will fail to persuade the hard-core group of confirmed skeptics who thrive on their own obstinacy. On the other hand, clear evidence of a change in the right direction of a response under carefully controlled laboratory conditions can markedly strengthen the case for the effectiveness of a drug or a procedure. This evidence is further enhanced if the scientific basis for the change is revealed.

A number of experiments in animals have been devised to try to settle these points, and although none of them gives unequivocal evidence that acupuncture does, in fact, have an analgesic action, the following are quite suggestive. In China, where a great deal of research has been done on this topic, some interesting experiments were witnessed by the U.S. study group in 1974. In one set of experiments, a beam of light from a heat lamp was focused on the nose of a rabbit, which was comfortably suspended in a cloth sling. The number of seconds that elapsed until the animal twitched its head away from the heat stimulus was recorded several times. When acupuncture was administered for 10 seconds before the heat stimulus was turned on, there was an increase of approximately 50 percent in the length of time the stimulus was tolerated in favorable instances. Acupuncture had a very similar influence on the tolerance to electrophoretic diffusion of potassium ions into the skin (i.e., potassium being charged positively can be driven across the skin under the influence of an electric current); this test produces quite pronounced pain and has been used frequently in human volunteers as a measure of threshold and tolerance to pain. An observation that was frequently made by Chinese investigators was that in at least 50 percent of experiments, acupuncture failed to modify tolerance to noxious stimuli.

Shortly after the first reports that acupuncture was being used successfully in China to control pain in humans, I decided, with a tongue-in-cheek attitude, that it would be of some interest to demonstrate that there was no scientific basis for such claims. At the time, we were doing some experiments in cats under general anesthesia; they consisted in stimulating one of the nerves supplying the skin of the face and recording the resultant discharge in that part of the sensory nucleus in the brain that is concerned with the relay of pain from the face. The discharge, called an evoked response, was recorded by means of electrodes applied to the surface of the brain stem at a point where the nucleus becomes superficial. The minute currents generated are amplified and displayed on a cathode-ray oscilloscope, an instrument that functions to some extent like the tube in a TV set in that it transforms electrical activity into a visible trace that can be observed and photographed. In this rather straightforward experiment, an evoked response of extremely consistent amplitude and shape can be readily obtained [Figure 12.2(*d*)]. The amplitude of the discharge is, up to a point, proportional to the intensity of the stimulus. The plan was to record the response characteristics photographically and then to see whether acupuncture stimulation modified it in any way. So convinced was I that no effect would be seen that it came as a complete surprise to see that after twenty minutes of electrical acupuncture stimulation delivered to the left forepaw, the evoked response was profoundly depressed [Figure 12.2(*d*)]. My immediate reaction was that the change had to be due to a failure in the recording technique. This conclusion was quickly proven to be wrong, since the response returned spontaneously and very gradually to normal over a period of six minutes. Furthermore, the effect could be obtained with identical characteristics time after time in that experiment. However, attempts to reproduce the phenomenon on subsequent days in other cats

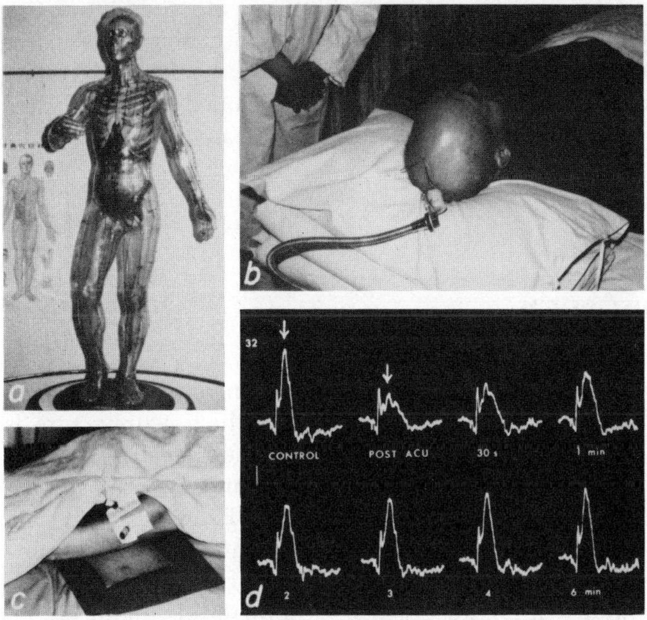

Figure 12.2. *(a)* The "meridians" used for acupuncture are shown in this plastic model and in charts on the wall.

(b) Mechanical acupuncture administered by electrically operated rotor.

(c) Moxibustion—patient's arm with needle holding smouldering moxa is shown.

(*d*) Pronounced depression of responses in a pain relay nucleus through twenty minutes of electrical acupuncture as described in text. Compare height of equivalent peaks before and after acupuncture (arrows) and recovery over a six-minute period.

Photographs (*a,b,* and *c*) taken by the author at the Peking Institute of Acupuncture and Moxibustion, Academy Traditional Chinese Medicine.

were entirely unsuccessful, despite the fact that the experiment was carried out in exactly the same way. Finally, on the seventh attempt, exactly the same result was again obtained; this total unpredictability of the acupuncture effect was characteristic of the long series of experiments that were carried out in an unsuccessful effort to determine the responsible mechanism. We could not conclude from this response that the relay of pain was being affected since, on one hand, the animals were always examined under general anesthesia and, on the other, innocuous sensations are also relayed through that part of the sensory nucleus. There was no doubt, however, that a very striking and unusually long-lasting phenomenon was occurring, and a guarded presumption was ventured that pain mechanisms might well be inhibited by it.

An important observation made at that time was that the effect could be obtained only from the deep tissues—that is, with the stimulating needle introduced into the muscle, as is the case in acupuncture in the human—but never from stimulating the skin itself. Especially interesting was the fact that once the acupuncture effect was obtained, it could elicited from a variety of sites, none of which were related to anything resembling a meridian.

ACUPUNCTURE FOR NONPAINFUL DISORDERS

There remain to be considered the far larger group of medical disorders and problems that are not primarily painful, but for which acupuncture is advertised as a cure. What should we believe about these claims? It should be remembered that acupuncture was used for thousands of years specifically for liver, kidney, cardiac, and other complaints. Examples of this are shown in Figure 12.2(*b*), in which acupuncture stimulation is being administered for paralysis resulting from a stroke; and in Figure 12.2(*c*), in which moxibustion is being given for treatment of a nonpainful condition.

The evidence here is completely anecdotal and unreliable, and there appears to be no reason to believe that the procedure is of the slightest value. This comment is not to be taken as a categorical denial that it does anything, ever, for disorders of the internal organs, since it is extremely difficult to produce evidence that any form of treatment is totally worthless under all circumstances. In fact, this very difficulty is the firmest basis on which quackery and cultist therapies of all types rest, assured that in a free society it is most difficult to prove beyond any reasonable doubt that what they purvey is anything but pure charlatanism.

What course should one follow, then, if one is afflicted with some chronic disorder of the liver, or other internal organ, for which no cure is yet available and one is advised to take a course of acupuncture? The chances are a thousand to one that it will be time and money wasted. Ethical acupuncturists will, in general, refuse to treat conditions that they believe are not susceptible to their ministrations. The ideal arrangement, when in doubt, would be to agree in advance with an acupuncturist who is willing to treat such a condition that payment for services be contingent on obvious improvement in signs or symptoms. Should, then, such agreements be extended to all practitioners of the healing arts? I shall not pursue the matter further, but leave the readers to draw their own conclusions on this score!

To conclude these comments on acupuncture for nonpainful problems, the method has been advocated for the cure of several types of addiction, ranging from smoking to alcoholism and even to dependence on heroin and other narcotics. Once again, there is no reason whatsoever to consider that acupuncture has anything to offer in these conditions, and those who make such claims are either totally misguided or perpetrating a hoax on the victims of these disorders. Similarly, bizarre types of acupuncture such as placing a metal clip on the earlobe or elsewhere have no more value than the incantations of shamans and witch doctors.

REFERENCES

Acupuncture analgesia in the People's Republic of China. Kaada, B., et al. *Tidsskr. Nord. Laegeforen* 94: 417–442, 1974

Acupuncture anesthesia. A translation of a Chinese publication of the same title. John E. Fogarty Center, Dept. of H.E.W. U.S. Govt. Printing Office, Publ. No. 75-784, 339 pp.

Acupuncture anesthesia in the People's Republic of China. A trip report of the American Acupuncture Study Group. Washington, D.C.: National Academy of Sciences, 1976

BONICA, J.J. Acupuncture anesthesia in the People's Republic of China: Implications for American medicine. *JAMA* 229: 1317–1325, 1974.

KATZ, R.L.; KAO, C. Y.; SPIEGEL, H., and KATZ, G.J. Pain, acupuncture and hypnosis. In: *Advances in Neurology* (Vol.4: 819–825). New York: Raven Press, 1974.

KERR, F.W.L.; WILSON, P.R.; and NIJENSOHN, D. Acupuncture reduces the trigeminal evoked response in decerebrate cats. *Experimental Neurology* 61: 84–95, 1978

13

Hypnosis and Biofeedback

The induction of trancelike states of consciousness in humans has been referred to since antiquity, but the first individual to make a detailed study of the phenomenon was Franz Anton Mesmer (Figure 13.1).

Over the years since Mesmer's experiences, more or less spectacular claims were made for hypnosis, not the least of which was that it could be used to relieve or abolish pain during surgical procedures; the great significance of this claim in the period prior to the discovery of anesthesia can well be imagined. Why hypnosis was not far more widely used as an analgesic at that time will become clear shortly, but that it was employed with signal success in many instances is well documented.

An early example of its use during an operation was reported in the *Bulletin of the Academy of Medicine of Paris* (Vol. II, page 370, 1829). The patient was a sixty-four-year-old woman who had cancer of the right breast that caused her much pain and loss of sleep. Her physician, a Doctor Chapelin, had found that she was quite responsive to "mesmerism" and had used this to relieve her pain. It then occurred to him that the tumor itself might be removed painlessly while she was under hypnotic suggestion; he arranged, therefore, with Professor Cloquet, a noted Parisian surgeon of the period, for the operation to take place on Sunday, April 12, 1829.

When M. Cloquet arrived at the patient's home, she was already sitting in an armchair in a hypnotic trance, with Doctor Chapelin supporting her right arm. An incision was made running from her axilla to her breast, and the tumor together with the involved lymph nodes was removed. During this procedure, the striking feature was the absence of any

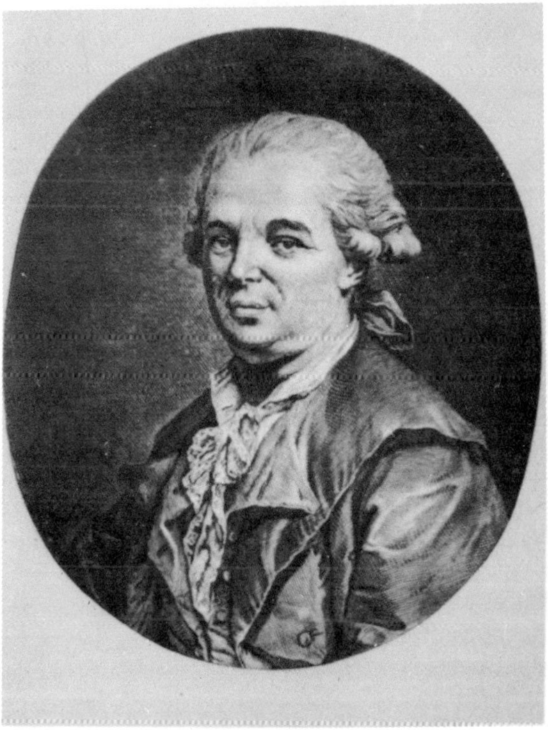

Figure 13.1. Franz Anton Mesmer (1734–1815).
The third of nine children, Mesmer was born at Iznang, a village near Lake Constance, Switzerland. After early education at religious schools, he entered the medical school at Vienna and was graduated in 1766. Marriage to a wealthy widow in 1768 relieved him of the burdens of earning a livelihood and gave him the opportunity to explore the phenomenon of hypnosis. He claimed that the universe was pervaded by a magnetic fluid with healing properties that he called "animal magnetism" and that he could channel into the bodies of others by laying his hands on them. His penchant for the theatrical brought him many patients and the enmity of his colleagues in Vienna. The latter circumstance led to his departure and relocation in Paris in 1778. Here his success was even greater, and he rapidly acquired a huge and devoted clientele, many of whom were of the aristocratic and moneyed classes. In order to attend to the large crowd who came for treatment, he devised a "magnetic tub" in which a number of patients could be treated simultaneously. Skepticism about Mesmer's unorthodox methods and reported cures led to the appointment in 1784 of a Royal Commission, one of whose members was Benjamin Franklin. The report of the commission was highly unfavorable, and although it recognized that a number of cures had indeed occurred, it attributed them to some as yet unidentified physiological phenomenon and ruled out any role for "magnetism." As a result, Mesmer's methods fell into disrepute, and shortly thereafter he retired to Switzerland, where he spent the remainder of his days. It appears that Mesmer sincerely believed in his methods and interpretations and that the charge of charlatanism is unjustified in his case.
Illustration courtesy of *Die Berühmte Arzte, 1967.*

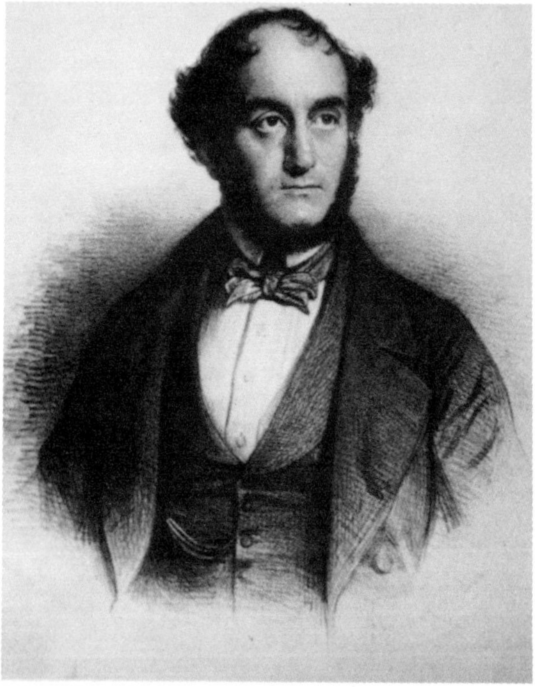

Figure 13.2. John Elliotson (1791–1868).
Elliotson was born in London, studied medicine at St. Thomas's and Guy's Hospitals, and took his M.D. degree in 1821. By nature a nonconformist, he discarded knee breeches and silk stockings, the customary dress of physicians of his day, and was one of the few who wore a beard. A man of outstanding intellect, he was appointed Lumleian lecturer (1829) and Professor of Clinical Medicine (1831) at London University and became President of the Royal Medical and Chirurgical Society of London.

His inquiring mind led him into areas frowned upon by his colleagues. Thus, he early became interested in phrenology and subsequently devoted much of his time to mesmerism. Because of the notoriety often associated with the latter, he incurred the displeasure of the Council of University College, from which he was forced to resign in 1838. Despite this, he continued his investigations on mesmerism and conducted frequent, well-attended séances at his home. He published his *Principles and Practices of Medicine* in 1839 and received the high distinction of being the Harveian orator in 1846. His more esoteric pursuits reflected neither on his character nor on his excellence as a physician, being regarded as the foremost in his profession. Thackeray dedicated *Pendennis* (1850) to him as a tribute to his skill, and Dickens also held him in high regard.

Illustration reprinted by permission from *Journal of the Royal College of Physicians of London* 6: 275, 1972.

signs of pain. To quote from the published report: "During all this time the patient continued to converse tranquilly with the operator, and gave not the least sign of sensibility. No movement in the limbs, nor in the patient's features, no change in the respiration or in the voice, and no changes in the pulse were observed." The hypnotic trance was maintained for forty-eight hours, during which time the wound was cleansed and dressed without any signs of suffering. When the patient was aroused from her trance, she was greatly agitated on finding that she had already been operated on and was again hypnotized as a means of tranquilizing her.

Cloquet reported the proceedings to the Academy of Medicine and was acrimoniously attacked by the noted surgeon Lisfranc, who refused to accept his testimony, inferring that Cloquet was either naive or mendacious.

Meanwhile, a number of distinguished English physicians became interested in mesmerism, as described in an excellent review by Hollander (1931–1932), from which some of the following accounts are taken. Mesmerism's most enthusiastic and scholarly advocate in that country was Dr. John Elliotson (Figure 13.2). Alarmed by Elliotson's espousal of mesmerism, his friends attempted, to no avail, to dissuade him from following what they believed to be a foolhardy course, due no doubt, to a temporary aberration in judgment. His detractors, however, delighted in the opportunity to revile him. Undeterred, he applied the method to a large number of patients and published his observations in a monograph (1843) entitled *Numerous Cases of Surgical Operations Without Pain in the Mesmeric State.*

Among the cases he described was that of a forty-two-year-old laborer who was suffering excruciating agony from an ulcerated knee joint. His leg was amputated on October 1, 1842, while he was under mesmerism administered by Mr. W. Topham, a barrister. The following account of the procedure, quoted by Hollander, is taken textually from Elliotson's monograph. "The placid look of his [the patient's] countenance never changed for an instant; not a muscle was seen to twitch. To the end of the operation, including the sawing of the bone, securing the arteries and applying the bandages, which occupied, in all, a period of upward of 20 minutes, he lay like a statue." After the operation he "gradually and calmly" awoke. After looking around, he exclaimed: "I bless the Lord to find it all over." He confessed that he had not felt any pain at all. He was again mesmerized for the first dressing of the wound. "Within 24 hours after the operation he was singing. In three weeks he sat up for dinner, and had not a single bad symptom." The case was reported at a medical meeting and, as summarized by Hollander, the following reactions occurred.

> No sooner had this paper been read, than up rose Mr. Coulson, a surgeon, who exclaimed: "This paper ought never to have been read; for the only

> point of interest was the non-expression of pain, and that was a common thing, and he had no doubt the man had been trained to it." At the following meeting of the Society it was proposed by Doctor Copeland to expunge the record of the meeting, for, he contended that: "If the account of the man experiencing no agony during the operation was true, the fact was unworthy of their consideration, because pain is a wise provision of nature, and patients ought to suffer pain while their surgeon is operating; they are all the better for it, and recover better." The motion was seconded by Doctor Evans and agreed to.

Despite these setbacks, reports of such striking control of pain during operations encouraged others to try the method in their medical practices. Among their number was James Esdaile (1808–1859), surgeon and Chief Medical Officer of the East India Company's hospital at Hooghly, Bengal. Professor Allan Webb of the Medical College of Calcutta visited this hospital on October 15, 1846, to see for himself whether the reports of painless surgery being performed there were based on fact or were simply idle gossip. When he arrived, the patients had already been hypnotized and were lying peacefully in bed. The surgeon proceeded to remove large tumors and excise ulcers from these patients without them envincing the least sign that they had been so much as touched. As Professor Webb stated, "Had they been sensible, this would have been torture so excruciating that the whole hospital would have rung with the shrieks of the patients." Referring to similar operations done in those days, he remarked: "I have seen many with the cold sweat of agony bubbling up for hours afterward, and a pulse so depressed that it was hazardous to move them, whereas these patients were quite chatty and lively."

Esdaile summarized his experience in two monographs entitled *Mesmerism in India* (1846) and *The Introduction of Mesmerism as an Anesthetic and Curative Agent* (1852). He used mesmerism to control pain in hundreds of operations, including amputations of limbs, hernias, stones in the bladder, amputation of the penis, cataracts, and for removal of many huge scrotal tumors caused by elephantiasis—all without losing a single patient during or immediately after the operation.

One may well ask, in view of these striking observations, why did hypnotism not rapidly become a standard procedure in all operations? Among reasons that can be cited, the skepticism and, it must be admitted, the overt callousness of some of the leaders of the medical profession played an important role. In France, if a physician was reported to be using mesmerism to treat patients, he was "struck off the register"; and in England, the Council of University College Hospital, London, prohibited its practice in their institution, a resolution that led to Elliotson's resignation from the staff.

Some of the opinions expressed by leading figures of the day are hard to reconcile with current attitudes toward pain. Magendie, the great French physiologist, is reported to have said that "pain was useful" and that he "doubted that there was any advantage in making patients insensible during an operation," adding that "it was a trivial matter to suffer, and that a discovery, the object of which was to prevent pain, was of little interest."* One may recollect similar opinions expressed by Copeland and by Lisfranc, as noted in previous pages.

However, the demise of mesmerism at that time as a method for controlling pain during surgery was undoubtedly brought about by the introduction of general anesthesia in 1846 (see Chapter 9). Liston's caustic comment that "ether anesthesia beats mesmerism hollow" (Chapter 9) indicates that not only was he familiar with hypnosis in this connection but also that it must have had serious shortcomings. In the intervening years up to the present time, hypnosis has had a somewhat checkered career.

Thus, it underwent a marked revival in France toward the end of the nineteenth century, when Jean Martin Charcot (1825–1893), the leading neurologist of his time, devoted considerable attention to its role in hysteria. He believed that hypnosis was a hysterical phenomenon, though his contemporaries and successors showed that it was readily demonstrable in normal individuals. Cycles of rejection and revival have continued to the present day.

One of the persistent problems that has dogged hypnosis in the treatment of pain is the belief that it is a subject fit only for the music hall or magician and, therefore, that it is inappropriate for consideration by practitioners of conventional medicine and related disciplines. This is unfortunate and stems from a lack of information regarding its usefulness; in some carefully selected pain problems, it can be more effective and useful than analgesic drugs, which provide only partial and brief relief of pain.

The fact that both the American and British Medical Associations now recognize hypnosis as an acceptable method of treatment that may be taught to medical students should reassure those who might otherwise continue to harbor serious reservations about the propriety of prescribing it.

CONTEMPORARY VIEWS ON HYPNOSIS

It is of considerable interest to try to assess, insofar as possible, what hypnosis itself is and under what circumstances it may be of value in the control of pain. The induction of a hypnotic state can be achieved in a

*Quoted by Hollander, *British Journal of Anaesthesiology,* 9: 1931–32.

number of ways. A common method requires the subject to look fixedly at a small ball suspended from a string while the hypnotist encourages him or her to relax and become drowsy. After a few minutes, the subject's eyelids droop and then close. At this point the suggestion may be made that some part of the body is either not felt or feels no pain. When the indicated area is then subjected to a painful stimulus, the subject gives no overt sign of discomfort and proceeds with his or her thoughts as if nothing were happening. This behavior raises the question of whether pain is being felt and attention is in some way diverted from it or whether for some other reason no complaint is made. If the hypnotic state is discontinued, the subject has no recollection of pain; this in turn raises the possibility that pain was felt at the time but that the memory process was somehow impaired.

Some of these interesting questions appear to have been resolved in experiments carried out by E. R. Hilgard of Stanford University, California, with strongly hypnotizable volunteers in whom the technique of automatic writing was used in an effort to uncover aspects of the subjects' inner experience that they could not communicate verbally (Hilgard and Hilgard 1975).

In automatic writing, the hand performs without the subject being aware of what is happening, or—as described by Hilgard—it is "out of awareness." In this manner a written record is obtained of a part of the subject's inner experience of which he or she is not aware but that is, nevertheless, very real. Using this technique, as well as a simpler method of automatic talking, Hilgard found that the volunteer subjects being tested for pain responses appeared to have two separate compartments in their consciousness. One of these, the hypnotized or "overt" part—the one that responded to questions in the usual manner seen in hypnosis—felt no pain. However, if the subjects were asked during hypnosis about the possibility that some part of their consciousness might be receiving painful messages, they were able to recall, when released from the hypnotic state, that, indeed, there had been such stimulation but that it had been much less distressing than equivalent pain without hypnosis. This second compartment of conscious experience was named "the hidden observer," and the sensation was designated as "covert" pain. Hilgard has noted that William James, as long ago as 1889, had postulated that there was evidence for "split consciousness" during hypnosis; these contemporary experiments give support for the concept.

Some General Facts Regarding Hypnosis

It is common knowledge that whereas some people are easily "hypnotizable," others are quite resistant or completely refractory to it. Less well known is the fact that no one can be hypnotized against his or her will and that cooperation by the subject is always necessary. Even with apparently full cooperation, there is a wide range of variability in the intensity of the hypnotic state that can be induced from person to person and, to some degree, within the same individual from one time to another. In a review of this topic, Hilgard concluded that 10 percent of the population cannot be hypnotized, that 30 percent develop a "drowsy-light" level of hypnosis, and that some 30 percent reach a moderate level. The remaining 30 percent enter the deep, trancelike state commonly thought of in connection with hypnosis.

Some individuals resist being hypnotized because they fear that they may be induced to say or do things that, under normal circumstances, they would refuse to do. However, hypnotists appear to be quite unanimous in denying this possibility; according to them, it is impossible to induce a patient under hypnosis to perform any act contrary to the subject's wishes or ethics.

What Do You Feel When Hypnotized?

Most people who have not been hypnotized believe that the subject who is deeply hypnotized is in a sleeplike state. However, T. X. Barber, a leading authority in the field, described his own experience as follows:

> In fact, when I am responding to test suggestions (while under hypnosis), I do not feel that my "state" differs in any important way from the state I am in when I watch a motion picture or a stage play. When I am in the audience, I let myself imagine and think with the communications from the stage, and I empathize, laugh, feel sad, cry and have other emotions, feelings and vicarious experiences that the actors are attempting to communicate.*

Yet when the subject receives a hypnotic suggestion that pain will not be felt in a certain area, and despite there being full consciousness as already described, there is no evidence whatsoever of discomfort, even when intense stimulation such as cutting or crushing is delivered.

Current Use of Hypnosis for Pain Relief

A point to keep in mind is that the effectiveness of hypnosis in pain control is directly proportional to the hypnotizability of the subject, though even highly hypnotizable subjects may fail to obtain pain relief. Since, as noted

***New York Times Magazine*, November 26, 1978. "Health—Coping with Pain through Hypnosis," by Spencer Klaw. © 1978 by The New York Times Company. Reprinted by permission.

earlier, only about 30 percent of the population develops a deep, trancelike state, it can be anticipated that not more than about one in three or four potential candidates for treatment of pain can be benefited.

A few of the areas in which hypnosis has been successful and some of the reasons for considering a trial of this method of treatment follow.

Surgery. Although major operations have been carried out under hypnotic suggestion without the subject showing or complaining in the slightest of pain, as described earlier in this section, there are few if any indications for its use in current operative practice. Anesthetics in the hands of expert personnel guarantee not only freedom from pain during the operation but also immobility of the patient and predictability of a good result throughout. In some cases of drug incompatibility or in those rare instances when anesthetic drugs are not available, hypnosis could be considered as an alternative method of anesthesia.

Obstetrics. The very wide range of responses according to personal and social attitudes toward childbirth and pain makes evaluation of analgesics in this setting somewhat more difficult than usual. Briefly, there are numerous published reports of deliveries being carried out under hypnosis with satisfactory control of pain, but the method is seldom used because in current obstetrical practice, adequate pain control can usually be obtained by standard methods. However, there are many women who would not agree at all with this last statement, often for very good reasons, in which cases hypnosis may be considered.

Dental Procedures. Here, again, very painful procedures such as drilling and extractions can be performed on a small proportion of carefully screened subjects without pain or with only minor discomfort. However, usual anesthetic measures are now so simple and predictably successful that there is little reason to resort to other methods.

Chronic Pain. The almost endless variety of causes and manifestations of chronic pain, whether due to cancer, arthritis, injury to nerves, or other sources, makes it quite impossible to deal in any depth with hypnosis in this context. Can any general rules be suggested for using hypnosis in a case of chronic pain? Perhaps one of the most cogent responses to this question has been given by Orne, who has had extensive experience in treating pain. He concludes (1980) that "if the patient happens to belong to the approximately 20% of the population who have the skill of experiencing profound hypnotic phenomena, there is good likelihood of almost complete relief." He also notes that in less hypnotizable or even unhypnotizable subjects, a variable and sometimes quite significant degree of relief can be obtained through hypnosis because of the placebo effect that it includes. For these and other reasons, such as its complete safety and ease of administration and because it is not habit-forming, he advocates at least a trial period of hypnosis in patients with chronic pain before considering surgical or other more aggressive procedures.

There are a number of reliable organizations in the United States that will provide information on hypnotists who are qualified to treat pain problems; among these the following are suggested:

Society for Clinical and Experimental Hypnosis
250 West End Avenue
New York, New York 10023

American Society of Clinical Hypnosis
2400 East Devon Avenue
Des Plaines, Illinois 60018

American Psychological Association
Division of Psychological Hypnosis
1200 17th Street N.W.
Washington, D.C. 20036

A RELATIONSHIP BETWEEN ACUPUNCTURE AND HYPNOSIS?

As one reflects on the peculiarities of acupuncture and hypnosis, certain similarities in the reactions of subjects to these two apparently very different procedures will be noted. For example, only about 20 percent of the population can be deeply hypnotized, and around 15 percent or somewhat less respond well to acupuncture for pain; is this the same group of people in both cases? If, furthermore, one remembers that the placebo effect accounts for around 20 percent of the relief of pain obtained by almost any procedure, it seems natural to wonder whether there is not a unifying theme in the background. Could it be that both acupunctural and hypnotic relief of pain can be attributed to the placebo effect?

In the case of chronic pain, the placebo effect may indeed play a very significant role, and it is often extremely difficult to decide how much of the relief of pain is due solely to this. On the other hand, in pain of a more acute nature and especially when it is severe—as in that associated with operations—even if the placebo effect is responsible for perhaps 20 to 30 percent of pain relief, it is highly unlikely that it could account for the profound "analgesia" that is such a striking feature when acupuncture or hypnosis is successful.

A major part of the pain relief must therefore be due to something other than placebo effect, but what is it? One possibility that has received considerable attention is that acupuncture "analgesia" is due to unintentional hypnotic influences. Katz et al (1974) found that patients who respond poorly to hypnotism almost invariably fail to obtain pain relief from acupuncture; they concluded therefore that they were probably dealing with parallel phenomena rather than an identical mechanism, but recognized that further studies would be necessary to reach more definitive conclusions.

BIOFEEDBACK

Biofeedback has become very popular as a result of extensive coverage by the media. It consists in a process of training the individual to assume better control over voluntary muscles, and in some instances, the involuntary uses of the blood vessels. One way of accomplishing this is to record the activity of the affected muscle by means of an electrode and then to amplify and display the electrical activity on an oscilloscope so that the subject has a visual representation of what is occurring. In the case of voluntary muscles that are in spasm and producing pain, the subject is able to see how the activity increases or decreases as he or she becomes more or less tense. Over a series of sessions, the individual learns to decrease the activity by relaxing and making positional or other adjustments. As he or she becomes more adept at this, the pain will tend to decrease. Similarly, when blood pressure levels and heart rate are visually displayed in this manner, some subjects are able to decrease either or both as a result of practice; in other words, an involuntary system comes under the control of the subject's will.

How Effective Is Biofeedback?

In cases of severe pain, it is probably of little value; at the present time its effectiveness for control of chronic pain remains to be demonstrated. As with other methods of treatment, it is very difficult to determine the degree to which suggestion (in its various forms—placebo effect, hypnotic suggestion) contributes to the successes claimed.

REFERENCES

BARBER, T.X. *Hypnosis: A scientific approach.* New York: Van Nostrand Reinhold, 1969.

ELLIOTSON, J. *Numerous cases of surgical operations without pain in the mesmeric state; with remarks upon the opposition of many members of the Royal Medical and*

Chirurgical Society and others to the reception of the unestimable blessings of mesmerism. Philadelphia: Lea & Febiger, 1843, 56 pp.

ESDAILE, J. *Mesmerism in India, and its application in surgery and medicine.* London: Longman, Brown, Green & Longmans, 1846, 287 pp.

ESDAILE, J. *The introduction of mesmerism as an anaesthetic and curative agent into the hospitals of India.* Perth: Dewar and Sons, 1852, 46 pp.

FORDYCE, W.E. *Behavioral methods for chronic pain and illness.* St. Louis, Mo.: C.V. Mosby, 1976.

HILGARD, E.R., and HILGARD, J.R. *Hypnosis in the relief of pain.* Los Altos, Calif.: Wm. Kaufmann, 1975, 262 pp.

HOLLANDER, B. Hypnosis and anesthesia. *British Journal Anaesthesiology* 9: 99–123, 1931–32.

KATZ, R.L.; KAO, C.Y.; SPIEGEL, H.; and KATZ, G.J. Pain, acupuncture and hypnosis. In *Advances in Neurology* (Vol. 4: 819–825). New York: Raven Press, 1974.

ORNE, M.T. Hypnotic control of pain: Toward a classification of the different psychological processes involved in pain. *Res. Pub. Assoc. Nerv. Ment. Dis.* 58: 155–172, 1980.

Glossary

AFFERENT: Carrying or conducting toward; thus, an *afferent* impulse travels toward the center being discussed.

ANALGESIA: The selective suppression of pain with preservation of consciousness and of other forms of sensation such as touch and pressure.

ANESTHESIA: Suppression of all sensation; if consciousness is lost in the process, it is termed *general anesthesia.* If consciousness is preserved, such as when a nerve is "blocked" with procaine, *local anesthesia* is said to have occurred.

AXON: The nerve fiber; it arises from the nerve cell or neuron and conducts messages away from it to other neurons.

BOUTON: Also *bouton terminal;* the enlarged ending of an axon that contains the chemical transmitter that is released onto nerve cells to excite or inhibit them. Also *end bulbs, synaptic endings.*

BRAIN STEM: Portion of central nervous system that extends from the upper end of the spinal cord up to and including the thalamus.

CENTRAL NERVOUS SYSTEM: The brain plus the spinal cord.

CERVICAL: Refers to the neck, as in *cervical disk;* a disk in the neck.

DENDRITE: From the Greek *dendron*—a tree. The branching processes that arise from the neuron soma. They receive contacts from other neurons and funnel the resulting impulses to their parent soma.

DISK, INTERVERTEBRAL: The soft cushion of tissue between the vertebral bodies.

DORSAL ROOT: The bundle of nerve fibers that enter the dorsal aspect of the spinal cord conveying sensory impulses.

EFFERENT: Carrying or directed away from.

ELECTRODE (metallic): A needle made of steel, silver, or other conductor, usually insulated except for its tip. Many varieties are made to meet different needs. Recording electrodes are used to pick up electric currents within tissues. Currents can be delivered through an electrode either to stimulate or to destroy tissue.

FORAMEN: A channel or passageway.

GANGLION: A collection of nerve cells; usually employed to describe those in the peripheral nervous system (e.g., *dorsal root ganglion*).

HERNIATED: Abnormal protrusion or bulging.

INHIBIT: To suppress activity.

INTEGRATION or INTEGRATIVE ACTIVITY: The ability of centers in the central nervous system to receive a diversity of incoming signals, sort them out, and forward an appropriate summary to other centers.

INTRACTABLE: That which does not respond to treatment; *refractory* or *persistent.*

LUMBAGO: An outdated term that means low back pain or lumbar pain.

LUMBAR: The lower part of the back between the lowest rib and the upper border of the pelvis.

MESENCEPHALON: The upper part of the brain stem, just below and behind the thalamus.

METASTASIS: A tumor that develops at a distance from the original site through spreading tumor cells via the bloodstream or other pathway.

MICRON or MICROMETER (abbr.: μm): A unit of length used especially in light microscopy; it is 1/1,000 of a millimeter (the diameter of a human hair is 60 micrometers).

MODULATE: To modify, usually in the sense of depressing or decreasing activity.

MORBIDITY (operative): Complications such as pain, infection, hemorrhage arising from an operation.

MYELIN: The sheath or covering around axons that are larger than 1 micron in diameter. It is composed of tightly apposed layers of cell membrane that contain protein and large amounts of fatty substance. It provides electrical insulation for the axon, which is referred to as a *myelinated fiber.*

NERVE IMPULSE: Conducted activity along a nerve fiber that can be detected with sensitive instruments as a minute traveling electrical charge. This is the means used by the nervous system to signal from one point to another, both in the nerves and in the brain.

NEURALGIA: Pain in a nerve.

NEURON: The nerve cell—it is composed of a body (*soma*) and processes (*dendrites* and *axon*).

NOCICEPTIVE: This term, which means receiver of noxious information, is used in preference to the word *pain* to avoid a prejudicial position. It is not pain that is present in the skin or peripheral nerves, but only signals that damage is occurring. When these messages reach consciousness, they evoke the complex experience we call pain.

NOCICEPTIVE SYSTEM: The system of peripheral nerve fibers and central nuclei and pathways involved in the detection, transmission, and perception of damaging (noxious) stimuli.

NOXIOUS: Damaging, threatening, or producing destruction of tissue.

NUCLEUS: A group of nerve cells (*neurons*) in the brain, usually involved in a particular function. For example, the hypoglossal nucleus is a group of motor cells that give origin to the hypoglossal nerve, which runs to the tongue to activate its muscles.

PAROXYSMAL: An event of sudden onset that repeats itself in a brief, irregular fashion for a short period of time.

PLACEBO: A pseudomedication—for example, a tablet of starch—that has no pharmacological action. Used to evaluate how much of a subject's response is due to his or her belief in the effectiveness of a drug.

POTENTIAL (electrical): An electrical charge such that the "amount" of electricity at a given point is greater than at another neutral point (usually ground), against which it is compared.

REFRACTORY: Equivalent to *unresponsive.* Thus, a painful condition is said to be *refractory* to treatment when it cannot be alleviated. A neuron can be in a *refractory* period, at which time it cannot be made to fire.

RHIZOTOMY: Operation to relieve pain by cutting a sensory root.

ROOT, DORSAL: Bundle of nerve fibers entering the dorsal surface of the spinal cord carrying sensory messages.

ROOT, VENTRAL: Bundle of nerve fibers emerging from the ventral surface of the spinal cord carrying motor messages.

SALTATORY CONDUCTION: The manner in which a nerve impulse jumps from one node to the next; from the Latin *saltare*—to jump.

SCIATICA: An outdated term that was used to describe pain running down the back of the thigh and leg.

SOMA: Body; in the case of a neuron, it is the *cell body.*

STEREOTAXIC APPARATUS: An instrument that is used to guide an electrode into position in the brain using the three spatial planes and an atlas of the brain.

SYNAPSE: The zone of the contact (*junction*) between the endings of an axon and another cell. More generally, a zone of contact between any parts of two neurons across which activity is initiated.

SYNDROME: A group of symptoms and signs that, taken together, serve to characterize a disorder or disease entity. For example, throbbing, one-sided headache preceded by vomiting and visual disturbances is characteristic of migraine or a migrainous syndrome.

THALAMUS: The major sensory nucleus in the center of the brain.

VISCERA: The internal organs; hence *visceral,* or to do with the organs.

Index